The Art of
Conscious
Parenting

"This book has expanded my mind on what it means to be green. *The Art of Conscious Parenting* gives us a 'green parenting' ecosystem for our children that, if followed, will guarantee that our kids will thrive and not just survive."

J. Stace McGee, president, Environmental Dynamics,
consultant to the U.S. Green Building Council

"This book will help us return to a wisdom we all have in our very bones. When free of the often destructive messages we imbibe from our culture, conscientiousness and conscience become the keys to successful parenting, family life, and world community. We ignore these lessons at deep peril to ourselves and our children."

David H. Albert, author of *And the Skylark Sings with Me:*
Homeschooling and Community-Based Education

"*The Art of Conscious Parenting* shows that ancient wisdom on early nurturing experiences is corroborated by a vast range of contemporary scientific studies. With rampant family dysfunction, depression, violence, and other endemic ills traceable to morbid patterns of child-rearing, we cannot afford to ignore the exciting challenges posed by this compelling, thought-provoking, and loving book."

Rabbi Avraham Greenbaum, author of *Wings of the Sun:*
Traditional Jewish Healing in Theory and Practice

"Yet was I a son to my father,
tender and alone before my mother.
Then he taught me and said to me:
Keep my ways and live;
Acquire wisdom, acquire understanding.

"So says King Solomon, the son of King David. The Fines have given every reader the opportunity to acquire wisdom and acquire the understanding to choose life for their future generations."

Rabbi Isaac Vachmann, Temple Shalom,
Pompano Beach, Florida

"Jeffrey and Dalit Fine's book lends insight into the sacred art of parenting and the science that sheds light on our deepest bond. No subject could be more important."

Alex Grey, author of *Sacred Mirrors* and *Transfigurations*

The Art of
Conscious
Parenting

The Natural Way to Give Birth, Bond with, and Raise Healthy Children

Jeffrey L. Fine, Ph.D.,
with Dalit Fine, M.S.

Healing Arts Press
Rochester, Vermont • Toronto, Canada

Parent
649.1

Healing Arts Press
One Park Street
Rochester, Vermont 05767
www.HealingArtsPress.com

Healing Arts Press is a division of Inner Traditions International

Note to the reader: *This book is intended as an informational guide. It is not
to be considered as medical advice, opinion, or treatment. It should not be used
to treat a serious ailment without prior consultation with a qualified health care
professional.*

Library of Congress Cataloging-in-Publication Data

Fine, Jeffrey L.
  The art of conscious parenting : the natural way to give birth, bond with, and
raise healthy children / Jeffrey L. Fine, with Dalit Fine.
    p. cm.
  Includes bibliographical references and index.
  ISBN 978-1-59477-322-8 (pbk.)
  1. Child rearing. 2. Childbirth. 3. Parent and child. 4. Parenting. I. Fine,
Dalit. II. Title.
  HQ769.F38 2009
  649'.1—dc22

                                                                    2009026253

Printed and bound in the United States by Lake Book Manufacturing

10   9   8   7   6   5   4   3   2   1

Text design and layout by Virginia Scott Bowman
This book was typeset in Garamond Premiere Pro and Agenda with Bodoni
Oldface and Gil Sans as display typefaces

To contact the authors of this book, go to their website: theNewParenting.com

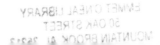

We dedicate this book to
The Blessed Holy One.
Our Endless Father-Mother-Creator
Who is Endlessly Fathering-Mothering-Creating
and
The Mothers and Fathers who will create
and parent all the future generations
and
Our son Kesem Joseph Fine whose
conception and life have been the
inspiration for this book

Contents

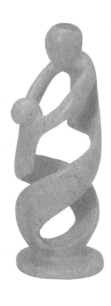

There's Nothing New Under the Sun

. . . there's nothing new under the sun.
Is there a thing of which it is said, "See this is new"?
It has already been, in the ages before us.

ECCLESIASTES 1:9

EVERY GENERATION THINKS THAT it is the first to discover the wonders of life: the joy of falling in love, the process of giving birth, and the pain and sorrow of loss. And yet we do not start over with each passing generation, we simply go in cycles. We rediscover the old wisdom, hopefully we make improvements, keep those things that are true and good, and disregard those things that just do not work. While the past cannot be idealized, it can certainly be a place to return to, in order to find answers and inspiration.

In the sixties, many young people moved toward a more organic approach to everything: from what they ate to how they gave birth; from how they used fossil fuel to what kind of natural fabrics they wore. This emerging generation seemed to be on a path to a more gentle existence reaching back to the simplicity of an earlier time. Somehow, between the times of college kids practicing nonviolent resistance to when video games became so violent that they could cause seizures in children, the practice of childbirth and child rearing changed dramatically. Somehow our society jumped back to the cold, sterile hospital practices of the fifties adding "new and improved drugs and technology," which won out over more natural rituals. Good parenting was defined by how many toys and electronic gadgets that Mom and Dad could buy for their young consumers. Now happily, Jeffrey and Dalit Fine have written a book about their journey to rediscover these "new" old ways and incorporate them into their lives and the life of their son. The obvious delight of just being with their child shines through on every page of this book. The profound experience of their son's birth has inspired them to teach and encourage others on how to follow this low-tech, natural approach to childbirth and child rearing.

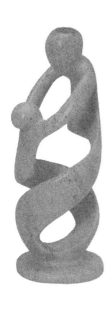

Not Just Another Book on Parenting

THERE ARE MANY BOOKS on parenting; library shelves bulge with them and a substantial number of them have landed, sooner or later, on my desk. Yet, in view of the rapid increase in the crisis of children affecting our nation, these literary efforts have had small effect.

Jeffrey and Dalit Fine's magnificent opus is different—indeed unique in all those crossing my path: and I have high hopes that this time, with his work, the vast bulwark of indifference such works have faced will be breached. I have rather lived with Jeffrey's work since its inception, or conception, a number of years ago, and while his first drafts seemed to hold promise, I had no idea of the scope, breadth, and depth there would be in this, the final result.

This book is far more than "just another book on parenting." It is an encyclopedia, a whole education in, and astonishing view of, the magnificent story of human conception, birth, and development. Nor am I just (or overly) prejudiced by his references to my own work. He has, at the very least, not just placed me in very good company, but thankfully has gone far beyond my own more cursory and tentative earlier surveys, updating them with the knowledge available today concerning the practices of birth-bonding and child-rearing; all of which knowledge is vast and magnificent and, within itself, the greatest story ever told or needing to be told.

Jeffrey's research and references, vast and valid, center on his current and immediate experience. My books were written largely after the fact of the ghastly birthing, broken bonding, and haphazard rearing of the first four of my five offspring. Looking back on the travesties of one's own stumbling past is both painful and enlightening. On the other hand, however, Jeffrey's insights are from his very current personal history concerning the comparatively recent conception and birth of his son. I stumbled into fatherhood and its ongoing series of exigencies and contingencies to be met as best one can. Jeffrey entered into the parent venture in an informed and intelligent manner, far more aware of what was at stake. His personal account of encounters with obstetricians and hospitals is both hilarious and sobering—a clear description of ill-informed medical interference, too often crass indifferences, and even stupidity.

It is my personal hope and prayer that now, as a result of Jeffrey's work and that of many others, far more people can be even more informed and prepared than either Jeffrey or myself. Our survival as a species may well depend on such revelation.

JOSEPH CHILTON PEARCE

For more than four decades, Joseph Chilton Pearce has been one of the seminal figures in the study of human consciousness and child development. He is the author of the groundbreaking *The Crack in the Cosmic Egg,* first published in 1971, which explores the nature of the mind and reality, and he later wrote several bestsellers on developmental psychology, including *Magical Child* and *Magical Child Matures.* In 2002 he published *The Biology of Transcendence* in which he examines how to move beyond the limitations of our current capacities of body and mind through the interaction of our brain with our heart, and in 2004 he coauthored, with Michael Mendizza, *Magical Parent Magical Child: The Art of Joyful Parenting.* He was a faculty member on childhood development at the Jung Institute in Switzerland and has taught at colleges and universities throughout the world about the changing needs of our children and the development of human society. Joseph Chilton Pearce is one of the visionary leaders of the twenty-first century.

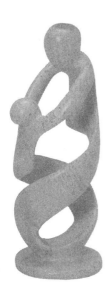

Don't Throw Your Baby Out with the Bath Water

AMERICAN WOMEN TODAY ARE facing a tragic loss. With the dominance of technological birth practices in the United States today, the American mother and child are being robbed of the simple and natural process of birth and bonding. Nature's organic program, built into the hard wiring of humans for millennia, has been disrupted and almost lost during the past seventy-five years.

A mother's ability to bond with her offspring during and after the process of birth is the most significant and essential characteristic of all mammalian females—especially human females—on this planet. This innate ability and the mother's knowledge that accompanies it have been so exploited, distorted, and trivialized by commercial thinking and conditioning that we no longer even see our loss.

We can certainly point to the results, however—even if we cannot always identify the cause:

- Men's and women's inability to connect in relationships at all levels
- Skyrocketing violence in our world
- The breakdown of consideration in the classroom

§ Rising rates of juvenile crime

§ Childhood despair and suicide

There are a number of studies that will be cited in the chapters to come, demonstrating the ways in which inadequate parental nurturing impedes growth of brain cells and alters a child's natural biology. What is important to understand at this point is the overall relationship between successful or unsuccessful maternal care, and between unsuccessful and successful child development. We know, for example, that:

1. Nature and the very force of evolution have placed a developmental template into every infant's central nervous system that is activated by quality maternal and paternal bonding. This template is designed to expedite the systematic and successful unfolding of an infant's physical, emotional, mental, and spiritual faculties.

2. A large portion of parents today, most of whom were raised at a time when the importance of bonding was unrecognized, raise their children in a way that ignores the cues and cries of the baby, and hence they unknowingly affect their child in inappropriate and harmful ways. This deprivation brings about hormonal, chemical, and physiological changes in the child's brain structure, and in his or her unfolding sense of self.

3. These changes, in turn, trigger psychological difficulties such as learning disabilities, hyperactivity, ADD-like symptoms, coping problems, aggressive tendencies, lack of impulse control, poor learning skills, inability to concentrate, and a catalogue of other misbehaviors.

4. The consequences of these misbehaviors can then become disastrous to the proper physical and mental growth of the child, as well as to the parents, to the family unit as a whole, and ultimately to society and the world at large. Whether caused by parental neglect, stress, indifference, inadequate knowledge, boredom, or any number of other factors, parents who fail to bond with their infant in an intimate way more or less guarantee, to some extent at any rate, a stunted child—and

thus a stunted adult. The saddest aspect of this unbonded childhood, moreover, is that it usually occurs not as a result of parental malice but largely because of ignorance, the pressures of modern life, and "expert" misinformation.

Scientific evidence points clearly to the destruction of the very fabric of our society if we do not restore birthing and bonding to the powers of the feminine.

This book helps to shed light on the path of this return. It is possible to return to the kind of birth that begins the process of creating and parenting human beings who can care for others and the world around them, use their creativity, and be strong in their understanding throughout their lives.

It all begins with *natural parenting* and the kind of birth that takes advantage of the fact that labor and delivery have been part of feminine knowledge for thousands of years, before the advent of the technology that so often plays an unnecessary role in birth today. We have written this book as a call to return to the kind of birthing and bonding that can play such an important role in the world to come.

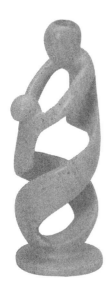

1

A New—or Old—Way to Think about Birth

The history of Western obstetrics is the history of technologies of separation. We've separated milk from breasts, mothers from babies, fetuses from pregnancies, sexuality from procreation, pregnancy from motherhood. And finally we're left with the image of the fetus as a free-floating being alone, analogous to man in space with the umbilical cord tethering the placental ship, and the mother reduced to the empty space that surrounds it.

It is very hard to conceptually put back together that which medicine has rendered asunder. . . . As I speak to different groups, from social scientists to birth practitioners, what I find is that I have a harder and harder time trying to make the meaning of connection, let alone the value of connection, understood.

BARBARA KATZ ROTHMAN, QUOTED IN *BIRTH AS AN AMERICAN RITE OF PASSAGE* BY ROBBIE FLOYD-DAVIS

RITES ANCIENT AND MODERN

A Chinese man walks to the graveyard one day. He is carrying a bowl of rice and vegetables that he intends to place on the tomb of his ancestors.

1

Along the way he meets an American.

"Why are you bringing all this perfectly good food to the grave-yard?" the American asks in a patronizing voice. "Your dead ancestor's can't taste."

"Perhaps," the Chinese man replies, smiling with an equal degree of condescension. "But I'll only answer your question if you first tell me why you Americans bring perfectly good flowers to the cemetery. As far as I know, your dead ancestors can't smell."

This tale shows that every civilization and every country has its own ways of dealing with the major life events that all of us experience from womb to tomb. Baptism, coming of age, marriage, last rites, death, burial: through these rites, all of us celebrate or mourn the human con-dition in ways that are distinctive to our culture's beliefs.

Of all the rites of passage we know of on the planet, perhaps none is practiced in a more diverse and intense way than the first and arguably the most important: birth and the child-rearing rituals that follow it.

Consider, for example, the way children are welcomed into life among the Ketchua Indians in Peru. Here a newborn is removed from the womb by three women who simultaneously hold the child's head, torso, and feet, chanting ancient tribal songs and making sacred hand gestures. They place the child directly on the mother's stomach, where it suckles and remains for the rest of the day. Part of the child's umbili-cal cord is then buried, and a tree is planted on the spot. From this moment on, the tree, representing heaven, and the cord, an embodi-ment of the child's eternal soul, are considered forever linked. In cer-tain tribes in Borneo newborns are delivered in total darkness so that disruptive psychic forces cannot infiltrate their spirit. At the moment of birth, herbal smoke is blown into the child's face by a shaman to cement the covenant between the infant and the breath of God. The mother and child are then placed in isolation for a day so that they can make intimate sensory acquaintance, learning to recognize each other's smell, sounds, expression, touch, and body signals.

Among the Laguna Pueblo Indians of the American Southwest,

parents bathe just-emerged newborns in a potion of yucca weed while prayers are chanted and songs of jubilation are sung. Just before the sun goes down, tribal elders paint the child's body with white clay. Believing that human beings are never more attuned to understanding the critical lessons of life than during the moments immediately following birth, the elders recite tribal wisdom into the little one's ear, simultaneously sprinkling ashes on the child's body as a reminder that we must all someday return to dust.

~

Compare these birth experiences to that in a society we know quite well: Mothers who are about to give birth are drugged, then wired to a bank of beeping, high-tech monitoring and hydrating equipment. Supine and with her legs spread before a group of strangers (most of them male professionals), the expectant mother finds herself in a bare, noisy delivery room beneath a heaven starred with blinding halogen lights. Technicians garbed in green scrubs mill around in obstetric masks, checking settings, tightening straps, watching as a male physician often pulls the newborn child out of the womb with an adjustable metal forceps or suction device. The child is then spanked smartly on the rear end to induce breathing, and the umbilical cord is cut and discarded without ceremony. After being scrubbed down with antiseptic detergent, and after fluids are vacuumed out the nose and mouth with a suctioning tube, the child has a brief visit with the mother before being whisked away from the mother's arms and breasts in order to be banded, vaccinated, fed artificially, and deposited in an isolated crib inside a room full of hundreds of other similarly birthed children.

Sound familiar? More than likely you and I were born in some version of this modern, industrial birthing ritual—not in a warm, dark, comfortable bedchamber surrounded by loving family and friends, but in a steel-framed hospital unit that smelled of antiseptic. This is the birth rite our particular society chooses for introducing newborns to the world. "Every society," anthropologist Gregory Bateson once remarked, "practices the birthing ceremonies that best mirror its values, norms, and philosophy."

But you might ask: Isn't this as it should be? Don't we believe, from centuries of trial and experience, that modern hospital delivery is the safest, fastest, and most hygienic form of childbirth?

Many people think so, certainly. Yet many others—a rapidly growing number, in fact—are beginning to realize that despite its sophisticated chemical and surgical procedures, modern obstetrics, with its uncompromising emphasis on technology over nature, comes up gravely lacking in the human arts. As many people are coming to understand, all children born under hospital lights and raised in a daycare-like environment end up being denied essential physical and emotional tools they need so profoundly to reach their full potential as human beings.

Regarding this lack of human arts in birth, neuropsychologist James Prescott reminds us of a fact that so many doctors and patients have forgotten, but that serves as a kind of battle cry for those who clearly see what is being done to both parents and children today. "No mammal on the planet separates the newborn from its mother at birth except the human animal," Prescott warns us. "No mammal on this planet denies the breast of the mother to the newborn except the human."[1]

Of course, in some instances where the health and well-being of the mother and/or child are greatly compromised because of physiological disease, diabetes, genetic difficulties, or other genuinely high risks, technological intervention can often save the life of both mother and child.

There's genuine trouble and the kind that is "manufactured."

But for you moms who have genuine medical problems and need medical supervision by all means get it. There are still many ways that you can naturally bond with your newborn and consciously parent him.

THE ART OF CONSCIOUS PARENTING

First, the bad news: This book is about the many adverse childbirth and child-rearing practices that have become the norm in our society—about the artificial disruption of essentially innate and self-guiding mammalian parenting processes. This book is also about the way certain high-tech obstetric and educational practices are not only medically unnecessary but also dangerous to the physical development and mental stability of our children. Also exposed here is the lack of awareness that many suffer from concerning the ways in which our inherent parental and biological rights have been stripped away from us by the very healing authorities we most trust, and how today these rights are denied parent and child routinely by a corporate-based, overly automated, and personally dehumanized technocratic system of obstetrics and child education.

This modern system, as many people are now coming to realize, ignores the first and most abiding of all medical principles: Do no harm. In the process, this system provokes fear and pain in parents, subjects mothers to unnecessary and sometimes dangerous medical and social practices, and in the end turns the delights of bearing and raising children into a science-fiction-style nightmare. Yet so persuaded are we today that the modern birthing model is the best model and, perhaps, the only model that we give this system our wholehearted confidence, approval, and gratitude.

But there's good news here too: this book is mostly about the methods that will remedy this situation by informing readers of a new body of remarkable scientific evidence that will help mothers avoid these dangers and, in the process, reestablish their faith in the million-year-old creative and healing powers of their own biological heritage.

Over the past several decades, this body of knowledge has been discovered or, more accurately, rediscovered by scientists and health care professionals working in a number of different medical, psychiatric, and therapeutic fields. These validated rediscoveries are being used to reeducate people concerning the real facts about childbirth and infant education. In the process, they are helping restore a fundamental human legacy to a society of parents that knows unconsciously that it has lost something dear—a society that cries out silently for a bodily wisdom it once so willingly gave away—and now so desperately needs to find again.

Both the theoretical and practical contents of this new knowledge are not based on New Age theories or anecdotal stories. Instead, they are derived from impeccable medical and cross-anthropological studies; from pediatric observation, academic study, and clinical practice; from double-blind trials and long-term surveys; from years of research mined in rarified scientific fields such as linguistics, neurobiology, and medical anthropology; and from the enormous volume of pooled experiential knowledge amassed by grassroots health care experts.

We call this combination of old and new wisdom the *new parenting*. Ironically, the massive amount of scientific data that has appeared in the past decades to support the growing movement of new parenting (also referred to as conscious parenting or attachment parenting) is as old as the human race. It is "new" only to us in the late twentieth and early twenty-first century who have been so mesmerized by technology that we have given up the biological practices that, for thousands of years, have activated normal intuition in parenthood and child raising. The new parenting is new, yes—but only to the contemporary Western world.

Yet, despite the rediscovery of child-rearing measures that have been part of world culture for eons, most of the ideas that drive the new conscious parenting remain little known and rarely practiced. Even when its most obvious and rudimentary principles are brought to the public's attention—when parents-to-be ask pediatricians about breastfeeding or water births; when subjects such as the dangers of birth-inducing chemicals or the premature cutting of the umbilical cord are brought up in the medical classroom; when psychiatric experts are questioned on TV talk shows concerning traditional child-rearing notions such as a child sleeping in the parents' bed or the importance of immediate eye contact between mother and newborn child; these ideas are usually dismissed with a raise of a professional eyebrow.

Indeed, it is not entirely paranoid to say that there is a silent conspiracy against many of the scientific principles, both stated and implicit, in the new parenting. Part of this conspiracy stems from simple prejudice, false information, and entrenched habits; but part is also based on more sinister reasons. Many of these new scientific findings, after all, are bad for profits. They do not sell enough artificial milk formula or cesarean sections to make them cost effective.

Yet in the process of sweeping aside the overwhelming amount of new evidence on the benefits of such practices as in-utero learning, natural birthing techniques, keeping mother and child together from the moment of birth onward, and much more, society is denied access to information that can dramatically lower the curve of childhood disease, childhood learning disabilities, juvenile violence, and willful self-destructiveness.

These negative behaviors, clearly evident in the anxiety-driven young people our society is producing in such numbers today, become increasingly common with every passing decade. If we look back just seventy or eighty years, we see that children rarely suffered from so many of the crippling problems that are such a common part of childhood's landscape today: chronic stress, learning deficits, hyperactivity, lack of concentration, autism, youthful eating disorders, preteen sexuality, alcoholism, drug use, childhood suicide, violently oppositional behavior, childhood crime, and even juvenile murder. These problems were rarely heard of and were often undreamed of in a gentler, less complex child-raising era.

The process of the new parenting suggests that many of these behaviors are a direct result of the flawed obstetric philosophies that separate mother and child, and more, that these behaviors can be reduced if not entirely reversed by returning to the old "new" ways of birthing and bringing up children.

BIRTHING, BONDING,
AND DOING IT OUR WAY

I practice nutritional medicine, I am a psychologist, and most important, the father of a son who is, at the time of the release of this book, ten years old.

In the mid-1980s, while living in New York City, I was introduced to a body of clinical studies that explored the science of early childhood development in new and entirely novel ways. Much of the most exciting and at times astonishing work in this area was written by a man named Joseph Chilton Pearce, author of the famous book *The Crack in the Cosmic Egg* and, later, of two bestsellers on developmental psychology: *Magical Child* and *Magical Child Matures*.

For a year or so I devoured every word of Pearce's work. The more I immersed myself in his thinking, the more I became convinced of its authenticity and stunning importance. At the time, I already possessed a solid grounding in child psychology from my own schooling and had done a fair amount of family counseling. In approaching Pearce's studies, I felt relatively well equipped to understand and assimilate his remarkable ideas.

What I was not prepared for was the urgent, even alarming seriousness of his message, of his willingness to oppose and contradict many of the "sacred cow" models of child raising that by now had become gospel in every doctor's office and home nursery; and of his insistence that if we do not soon take measures to remedy the way we birth and parent our children in this society, our very species will be endangered and ultimately will destroy itself along with the planetary habitat that surrounds it. Interestingly, today, twenty years after Pearce first wrote of them, we see that an alarming number of his predictions have come true.

Eventually I became so fascinated with this new body of knowledge that I sought out Joseph Pearce personally. After attending his lectures and after several personal conversations, I found him to be a welcoming and brilliant mentor. In the months that followed, I took several of his three-day workshops, sat in on his seminars, and held long conversations with him on a variety of topics, most of which were related to children, families, and the psychology of the human spirit.

In the process I became familiar with the canon of scientific evidence he had amassed. This information documented the fact that lack of bonding between mother and child is producing dire effects on the American mother's ability to become responsive to her children biologically and emotionally and that our psychology of the developing infant is based on flawed and outmoded nineteenth-century precepts that can be traced from Sigmund Freud to Dr. Spock.

Gradually, Pearce's studies began to have a noticeable effect on my own clinical technique as a psychotherapist and family counselor. I now started giving guidance to patients based largely on his research and on certain ideas formulated by his colleagues. I was a bit apprehensive at first, but the bread I cast on the waters soon returned in the form of clear evidence that my patients were parenting more effectively and nurturing their children better and that even the most deeply damaged family relationships were capable of being healed.

It was all very new and very heady work.

PRACTICAL APPLICATION

Over the years Joseph Chilton Pearce and I continued to stay in touch. His ideas became increasingly central to my work. As with everything, however, the glow of their newness faded as time passed, and they quietly took their place alongside the other healing modalities on my clinician's shelf. In my private world I was unmarried. Pearce's theories of child development, while clinically exhilarating, had little significance for my personal life.

Then, several years later, I met the love of my life: a beautiful young Israeli woman named Dalit, whom I wooed and married. We settled down in New York City, and after a year and a half, all that I had been reading about and studying became very real for me: my new wife became pregnant.

Given the fact that I was already a believer in Joe Pearce's galaxy of psychological, developmental, and biological ideas concerning childbirth; and given the fact that I had a great deal of experience in natural healing modalities, you might imagine that the moment I learned I was a father-to-be, I would return to Pearce's work and use it to birth and raise my own child.

This, however, was not entirely the case. Like so many prospective parents, the fearful warnings that had been branded into my unconscious by the medical profession since I was a young man echoed loudly in my head and in my wife's head like an apocalyptic litany. It cautioned that childbirth is a dangerous event. *Very* dangerous. So many mothers have died in the past: They hemorrhage to death; they succumb to infection. The child dies along with the mother. The situation is grave.

So we heard: Be wise and take all the medical precautions you can. Avail yourself of the latest surgical and chemical technology. Do not dream of delivering your baby anywhere but in a hospital delivery room—and never, ever allow your baby to be brought into the world by anyone other than a qualified obstetrician.

In the dark scenario of medical childbirth, these were the words of warning that had been imprinted on our brains. There were other words: *pain, exhaustion, defects in the fetus, sepsis, complications, blood, and death.*

But nowhere in the litany of cautions and disaster did either of us ever hear the word *joy*. We were appropriately intimidated and scared.

⁓

What is related in the following pages, beyond information based on much study, is what we learned and discovered—or rediscovered—in the process of birthing and nurturing our son. The chapters here—on the child's learning in the womb, on labor and delivery, on the importance of breastfeeding, and on raising whole, caring, strong human beings in the months and years after childbirth—beyond translating the facts that have been defined from years of research, also speak to our experience as parents who have engaged in all of it.

Here, you will find not just a method on a page, but a way that has worked for many for thousands of years—and for us, very regular people who began this process with the desires and concerns that any parents share.

We hope you will rediscover what we have learned as we've traversed this ground.

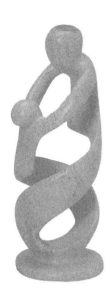

2

High-Tech Birth
and the Alternative

*"The greatest terror a child can have is that he is not
loved, and rejection is the hell he fears. I think everyone
in the world to a large or small extent has felt rejection.
And with rejection comes anger, and with anger some
kind of crime in revenge for the rejection, and with the
crime, guilt—and there is the story of mankind."*

JOHN STEINBECK, *EAST OF EDEN*

A MODEL BIRTH

"The way a society conceives of and uses technology," writes anthropologist, Dr. Robbie Davis-Floyd, "reflects and perpetuates the value and belief system that underlies it . . . and like all health-care systems, it embodies the biases and beliefs of the society that created it."[1]

Our Western society's core value system, Davis-Floyd points out, is oriented toward a scientific worldview that is sponsored in an undisguised way by large medical institutions governed by profit-driven medical ideologies.

Given this tendency towards a technological bias, our culture has as a matter of course developed a cyborglike model of the human body. In a mechanized philosophy that barely recognizes the intuitive and interior sides of man and woman, it is only natural that modern

11

medicine views human beings as sophisticated cyborgs that when ailing are best restored to their proper functioning by mechanistic interventions such as prescriptive chemicals and appropriate surgeries.

An unfortunate side effect of this mechanized view of the body and of medicine as an industrial trade is that many doctors now look on their profession not as a divine calling or even as a dedicated life work, but simply as "just another business."

I recall once speaking with a physician patient of mine whose son was due to graduate from college. I asked him what profession his son intended to follow.

"He's not sure yet," the doctor replied. "But he thinks it will either be law, business, or maybe medicine."

Maybe medicine? Like retailing or the legal profession? For many, it's just another business option.

Because the robotic prototype of the human body has become effectively the working basis of all modern medicine, it comes as no surprise that this same mechanistic metaphor has been carried over to the birthing room, where high-tech equipment and no-nonsense (that is, emotionally uninvolved) medical practitioners "cure" the female "patient" of her disorder: the "nine-month disease" of pregnancy.

Writes Floyd:

> As the factory production of goods became the central organizing metaphor for social life, it also became the dominant metaphor for birth: the hospital became the factory, the mother's body became the machine, and the baby became the produce of an industrial manufacturing process. Obstetrics was thereby enjoined to develop tools and technologies for the manipulation and improvement of the inherently defective process of birth, and to make birth conform to the assembly-line model of factory production.[2]

Never mind whether this assembly-line method of delivering newborns works well. Through years of jockeying and politics and finagling and brainwashing on the part of those who profit most from the medical model of birth, the hospital system is now a sacred norm. To suggest that there is a better, safer, kinder way of having a child is looked on by a majority of people as a heresy, an ingratitude towards the life-improving marvels of technology, and a suicidal return to the medicine of the Middle Ages.

Yet such an attitude is itself part of the cultural bias Davis-Floyd recounts. "As has been clear for over twenty years," she writes, "most routine obstetrical procedures have little or no scientific evidence to justify them. They are routinely performed not because they make scientific sense, but because they make cultural sense. They exemplify certain fundamental aspects of technocratic life."[3]

Who has the authority: pregnant mothers or the medical establishment? In her article "Authoritative Knowledge and its Construction"[4] in the book *Childbirth and Authoritative Knowledge: Cross Cultural Perspectives,* anthropologist and pediatrician Brigitte Jordan tells of investigating a legal case in which a group of pregnant American mothers were ordered by a judge and court of law during the late 1980s to give birth by cesarean section. Some of these women were insistent that they neither needed nor wanted this procedure. Others delivered their child surreptitiously at home or in hiding. Many were forced to comply.

Besides the Big Brother overtones of this ruling, and the denial of the procreative liberties we assume are every American woman's rights, what most amazed Jordan was the fact that after studying carefully the medical history of these cases, she concluded that not one of the cesarean operations forced on the women proved to be medically necessary. Following their own body wisdom and maternal intuitions, the dissenting mothers had been right all along.

"I began to think seriously about why and how it was the case that women's knowledge didn't count while medical knowledge carried the day," writes Jordan. "Which kind of knowledge was 'correct' obviously wasn't the decisive factor."[5]

Cesarean birth has, of course, become heavily politicized today, and some doctors and medical organizations, citing the "hygienic" and "safety" benefits of this procedure, are lobbying to make cesarean sections (c-sections) an optional choice for all pregnant American mothers. Never mind, as Michel Odent, one of the world's foremost scientific authorities on childbirth, warns in his book *The Caesarean*.[6] In the early to mid-twentieth century, before medical instrumentation took over the delivery room, the need for such surgical procedures was minimal. Statistically speaking, Odent reports, feedback from electronic fetal monitoring machines (compared simply to listening to the mother's heartbeat with a stethoscope) is often so undependable that many cesarean births not only prove clinically uncalled for, but also later end up creating physical complications for the mother, the infant, or both, that continue for years. The many hazards of this sometimes useful but often needless practice are profiled in the Birthing chapter further on.

Regarding Jordan's research, the notion that concerned her most in her studies—the forced c-sections in the legal case she investigated and in other, similar cases—was the fact that during labor and delivery in a modern hospital setting, every iota of power and self-determination is taken away from parents and handed over to the medical professionals, especially the obstetrician.

Jordan goes on to describe a typical birth experience of a twenty-five-year-old woman in her tenth hour of labor having her second child. The entire event was videotaped: Present in the delivery room were the pregnant mother, her husband, a nurse-technician, and a parade of other medical professionals. As is clearly displayed on this famous tape, the husband of the pregnant woman appears to be intimidated by his wife's helplessness and by the hospital staff. He approaches his wife's bedside when called, but scurries away when the medical team moves in.

The attending nurse, meanwhile, seems less concerned with her "patient" than with studying the oscillations on the electronic fetal monitor (EFM) screen. "The EFM is widely believed to give early warning of intrauterine difficulties," writes Jordan, "even though it has never been shown that routine EFM treatment improves birth outcome."[7]

Most significantly, when the mother begins to enter the second stage of labor and starts to undergo increasingly powerful urges to push that "become progressively more irresistible until the baby is finally pushed out,"[8] the nurse-technician, using stern warnings and infantalizing praise, insists that the woman not push until the doctor arrives. "Every effort is made to keep her from giving in to the overpowering impulse to bear down," writes Jordan. "She is asked to suppress the urge long enough for the physician to come in and pronounce her ready."[9]

The physician, however, is busy elsewhere. He is paged several times, but does not appear. Where is he? No one knows.

The nurse leaves the room to search for the doctor while a medical student and a nursing student replace her. This pair proceeds to perform a vaginal examination on the mother without asking her permission, and without explaining what they are doing or why they are doing it. "The examination is inconclusive both in the sense that the medical student cannot feel what the state of the woman's cervix is, and in the sense that even if she knew, it wouldn't matter because she cannot give the official permission to push."[10]

Finally, the doctor arrives accompanied by a coterie of male medical students who have come to watch the proceedings, though they are uninvited and unwanted by the mother-to-be. Without apology for his tardiness, and without a glance at his patient, the physician strides over to the fetal monitoring machine, peruses the data, and confers with several of his medical students. Then—speaking to the nurse, not the mother—he announces what the mother has already known for an hour, that she is ready to start pushing.

The pregnant mother's feet are now placed in stirrups and she is washed down with an antiseptic solution. The husband is told to take his place at the head of the bed. One of the medical students slips on a pair of surgical gloves while the physician stands nearby, holding a suctioning tube. As the newborn's head emerges, the doctor suctions out fluids from the baby's nose and mouth. The child is delivered by one of his medical students, not by the doctor himself.

Again, Jordan notes that not only is the expectant mother utterly unempowered at the very moment she should be making vital choices, overseeing the mechanics of her posture, contractions, and positioning; not only is the innate knowledge of her own body processes ignored by the medical professionals who surround her; but also her status as a feeling, thinking human being is completely minimized. Throughout the delivery the doctor rarely looks at his patient and does not converse with her at all. There's never an encouraging smile, never a kind word. It's all business.

> When the doctor finally allows that the patient can push, this announcement is directed to the medical team, not to the mother. The doctor says "She can push," and the nurse relays the message, "He says you can push," as if doctor and woman were not in the same room. In the ways in which the participation structure is set up in the labor room, her [the mother's] exclusion is ratified, executed, and displayed over and over again. This is one of the mechanisms by which she is denied any say in the conduct of her labor, by which she is given the message that she doesn't count.[11]

Yet while Jordan calls out against the harsh mechanization and alienation of a rite of passage that, under more humane conditions, would be surrounded with light and love, what disturbs her most is the fact that the mother-to-be—the one who is, after all, having the baby, and who senses the motion and inclination of the child within her—is barred from offering any input whatsoever concerning her feelings, her needs, her pain, observations, suggestions, and her own precious knowledge of what is actually taking place inside her womb.

The truth is that the doctors, medical students, nurses, and others, despite their shows of authority and expertise, have only a limited physiological knowledge of what is really happening to patient and child. The person who does know, meanwhile, is semi-abandoned by her intimidated husband; is reduced systematically to childlike status by the authoritarian cajoling of the nurse; has her womanhood exposed to the cold, clinical eyes of an uninvited group of male medical students; is ignored entirely by the grand panjandrum himself, the obstetric physician; and finally, adding insult to injury, after a brief post delivery hug session, she is forced to give over her newborn to the masked clinicians in the obstetric ward at the very time when this new little human being needs a mother's warmth, gaze, voice, coddling, and love more than at any other moment in its life. In the end, this controlled, belittled, and forgotten victim of the technical model of medicine is, as Jordan points out, "not giving birth; she is delivered."[12]

Joseph Chilton Pearce, one of the world's foremost writers on child development and new parenting methods, and a thinker whose ideas I will refer to frequently in this book, tells us in decidedly unequivocal terms:

> Hospital-medical childbirth now made sacrosanct and unquestioned on every hand is a more insidious and devious danger than atomic bombs or germ warfare, since unrecognized and even *unrecognizable* by the public at large for the demonic force it is. Taking away a woman's rights over her own reproductive process has been a disaster; but intervening and all but abolishing the bonding of mother with infant at birth is a devastating crime against nature; perhaps the most criminal and destructive act on the planet today, and an ultimate, if slow but sure, instrument for "species" suicide.[13]

A DISTURBING SURPRISE

In 1956, French physician Marcelle Geber traveled to the African country of Uganda to perform an urgent mission of mercy.

Uganda was a poor place in 1956, as it is today, and there was a great deal of fretting in the United Nations and other diplomatic circles that its people might not survive the rigors of the twentieth century. According to reports, malnutrition and disease were rampaging over much of central Africa like horsemen of the Apocalypse, taking a ghastly toll. The Ugandan per capita income was miniscule and growing smaller every year while the population was increasing at geometric proportions and unemployment was gripping almost half the country's workforce. Worst of all, rumor had it that Ugandan infants were being mistreated, and that many were dying daily from parental abandonment and neglect.

Geber set sail for Africa on a research grant from the United Nations Children's Fund, determined to save the children. Once on the continent, she spent a good deal of time both in Uganda and Kenya, studying the customs and culture there, making the acquaintance of a wide range of villagers, and observing the ways in which African parents birthed and raised their young.

The discoveries that Geber made were profoundly disturbing—but not because she found Ugandan parents failing in their duties: far from it. In this poor, undeveloped land, among an uneducated, technologically backward population, where children were born without modern medical care under the most precarious conditions—sometimes in the back of a tea shop or in the family hut—Geber witnessed newborns who were far more responsive, physically agile, mentally progressed, and emotionally adjusted than their infant counterparts in the West. In the words of Joseph Chilton Pearce:

> Geber found the most precocious, brilliant, and advanced infants and children ever observed anywhere. These infants had smiled continuously and rapturously from, at the latest, their fourth day of life. Sensorimotor learning and general development were phenomenal, indeed miraculous. . . . The Ugandan infants were months ahead of American and European children.[14]

These remarkable observations caused Geber to begin questioning her previous assumptions concerning the benefits of Western birthing techniques and Western child-rearing techniques in general. What caused this profound difference between the developmental graph of the African child and the Western child? She wanted to know.

As it turned out, there were a number of factors, many of them emotional, some purely physiological. During the hours of birth and delivery, for example, Geber knew that large amounts of adrenalin hormone circulate throughout an infant's system. This stimulating hormone is needed at the time of delivery to energize the newborn and expedite birth. If it remains in a child's system too long, however, it can trigger a range of anxiety-based disturbances. As it turned out, an analysis of blood samples taken from newborn Ugandan children showed that on the average all adrenal steroids connected with birth stress were absent from the children's systems approximately four days after delivery. As a result, Ugandan newborns were serene and relaxed and rarely suffered from colic.

Among modern, industrialized nations, on the other hand, a number of studies show that adrenalin levels remain elevated in a newborn's systems for several weeks and sometimes for several months after delivery. The damages incurred from the lingering presence of this stimulating hormone not only produces highly anxious children, but also it can return to haunt a person during adulthood in the form of depression, phobias, and other mental disorders.

Then there is the question of the birthing environment. Geber found from her fieldwork that most Ugandan children were born at home, aided by friends and family. In this primitive domestic setting, delivery took an hour or two at most and was, by all reports, virtually painless for the mother. Within a short period of time after the child was born, moreover, the new mother was on her feet and out the door, strolling around the village, talking to neighbors, and showing off her newborn child to local admirers.

Were people in the community surprised that this young woman had given birth an hour or so earlier and was now busily visiting friends? Not at all. This is the way a new Ugandan mother always proceeds.

Within a few days, what's more, these same infants would be starting to sit up straight, held only by the mother's forearms, a feat considered impossible in the West. The babes smiled frequently (how many parents recall their pediatrician's warning that a newborn's smile is really nothing more than "gas"?), and on occasion they gave tiny tinkle sounds that clearly resembled laughs. Unlike Western newborns, who sleep most of the time during the first weeks after birth, these children remained awake a majority of the day and were almost never cranky or out of sorts.

"These infants [in Geber's studies] were awake a surprising amount of time—alert, watchful, happy, and calm," writes Pearce. "They virtually never cried. The mother responded to the infant's every gesture, and assisted the child in every move that was undertaken, so that every move initiated by the child ended in immediate success. And they smiled and smiled."[15]

Here, it is important to note that African mothers by no means have a monopoly on placid babies and rapid postpartum recovery. Ease of birth and quickness of recovery ultimately have little to do with place and nationality; method is all. Our son's birth, as you will see, took place in a New York City natural birthing center, where approximately an hour after delivery my wife, Dalit, was walking our new baby son, Kesem, up and down the birthing room, basking in *ohs* and *ahs* from friends and relatives. In this age-old moment of ceremonial display, my wife could as easily have been making her circuit in a village square in India or Japan or Guatemala or, for that matter, anywhere on the planet.

She was able to recover from the efforts of childbirth so swiftly and to walk proudly with her new child not because she had any special powers, but because, like her Ugandan sisters, she had just given birth in an undisturbed, nondrugged state, untroubled by beeping monitors and chemical injections, and emotionally aided and physically supported by a loving husband and a wise midwife in a warm, low-light, quiet, and immensely caring birthing environment. The area was free of peeping medical students, authoritarian nurses, and imperious physicians. Usually, this is all it takes.

A similar positive child-rearing outcome derives from the age-old practice of keeping an infant "skin to skin" with the mother during the first few days and months after delivery. In her cultural studies, Geber made the discovery that from the hour of birth onward, Ugandan mothers carried their newborns around pressed tightly against their bodies in a cloth sling. Throughout the day, the mothers cuddled their nurslings—they talked to them, sang to them, smiled at them, and, most significantly, granted them on-demand breastfeeding.

In fact, during these early days of childhood, Ugandan mothers were seldom parted from their infants. Wherever they went, the child was in direct contact with the mother's body, lying dreamily against a warm wall of flesh just inches away from freely available milk-laden breasts. Whether at the marketplace, feeding the cows, cooking a meal, or even at work, mother and child were constantly and literally in touch. At the time Geber visited Uganda, it was not an unusual sight to see a female employee sitting at a desk in a modern office, typing away while her infant child sat on her lap and quietly nursed at her breasts.

Like the Ugandan mother, and like mothers throughout the more traditional parts of the world, my wife, Dalit, also kept our newborn son snuggled comfortably next to her body throughout the day as she went about her daily activities. In this skin-to-skin posture, my wife's breasts were always available to our son Kesem, serving as a source of nourishment, but also acting as a kind of magically poetic metaphor, making him feel as if he were basking in the warm and ever-secure "bosom of the world."

Interestingly, no one ever educated us in this skin-to-skin technique. We more or less stumbled on it instinctively. Indeed, as a result of going against the grain, we had the nagging sensation occasionally that perhaps we were doing something parentally "incorrect" or that we were somehow harming our child. One doctor friend of mine even warned: "You know, Jeffery, you want your child to become independent as quickly as possible. Don't mollycoddle him too much the way you're doing—even when he's a newborn. Otherwise you'll all become codependents; you and Dalit will never have any time for yourselves. Kesem will become so demanding and used to getting his way that he'll drive you crazy."

What we did not realize at the time was that within the borders of our society, where autonomy from parents is considered a kind of sacrament, most families consider the continual, loving contact of mother and child the very foundation of infant care. What we had done, in short, is what so many parents have tried to do down through the ages: we had used every means at our disposal to bond properly with our newborn child.

BONDING

More than a half century ago, the great German naturalist Konrad Lorenz discovered that if a human being voluntarily takes over the care and raising of a newborn jackdaw, the fledgling bird soon comes to look on the human keeper as its parent.

From the moment this light goes on in the baby bird's brain, an unbreakable attachment forms between the avian world and the human—one that cannot be broken and that will last a lifetime. Henceforth, the infant jackdaw will give itself over entirely to its surrogate human parents, waddling after them everywhere like a baby duck behind a mama bird, frolicking with them, mimicking them, and loving them exactly as it would its own jackdaw mother.

Lorenz dubbed this process *biological and social imprinting.* Over the years, the German biologist's theories found their way into common psychological practice, though his somewhat clinical term *imprinting* eventually morphed into the more expressive term *bonding,* a word that has today passed into the vernacular. We speak now of bonding with our teammates, with a favorite beer mug, or with our dog.

For psychologists, however, the term *bonding* is reserved exclusively for kinship relationships—specifically for relationships between mates and between parent and child. Any partnership or parental liaison whose central core depends upon a long-term, unconditionally loving commitment is a form of bonding. In its deepest manifestation it is a mysterious and indefinable link between souls. "Bonding," writes Joseph Chilton Pearce, "is a nonverbal form of psychological communication, an intuitive rapport that operates outside or beyond ordinary rational, linear ways of thinking and perceiving."[16]

Thus, the many remarkable behavior patterns that Geber observed while in Uganda could in some way be traced back to the bonding techniques practiced as a matter of custom and course by Ugandan mothers. As a number of scientific studies are now bearing out, the quality of such bonding is a major determinant of our behavior patterns as adults. Included on the list of behavior that is influenced by proper bonding—or a lack of it—are physical health, immune system strength, mental well being, learning skills, ability to socialize, and the capacity to love ourselves and other people.

Studies likewise show that the more dependent small children are on their parents during the first five to six years, the more independent these children grow up to be—not vice versa, as is so often assumed in our society. Indeed, in many psychologists' opinions, the all-powerful, highly complex human bonding between mother and child is the single most important determinant of a person's future creativity, strength of mind, emotional intelligence, and sense of self. Through the maternal relationship, infants receive their first impressions of the world. The mother's face is the first face they see, her voice the first voice they hear. When the child's virgin senses—taste, touch, smell, sight, sound—are played upon for the first time like five finely tuned musical strings, it is the mother who wields the bow. She is the infant's initial social contact, the primary inspirer of the child's feelings, the infant's first playmate, lover, role model, friend. She is the gateway through which the child's psyche and spirit pass into the physical plane, and ideally she is the guardian who prepares the young one for life in a difficult world.

Moreover, bonding, as a kind of eternity symbol that circulates love endlessly and effortlessly between parent and child, is also a biological imperative programmed into both human beings. This imperative has a strong genetic component: Neither mother nor child needs instructions on how to put it to work. It is designed by the manufacturer to be beneficial to both parties. In addition, it is meant not only to ensure that the infant succeeds, but also to ensure that the mother received continuous care, which, when we view it in the larger picture, becomes a survival mechanism for the human species itself.

In one famous pioneer experiment in bonding conducted in the 1960s, psychologist Harry Harlow* placed two mechanical chimp mothers in a cage with newborn chimps. One of the surrogate mothers was covered with wire, the other with soft terry cloth. The cold, steel-wire mother was equipped with a nipple for dispensing milk. The terry cloth-wrapped monkey mother offered no food at all—just softness and the warmth of the cuddly material.

As it turned out, though the wire mother was a source of food, the baby chimps spent most of their time nuzzling and hugging the soft cloth monkey. These findings led researchers to believe that higher mammals'—including humans'—need for closeness, warmth, comfort, and affection is as important to infants as the need to be fed. In his famous address at a convention of the American Psychological Association, Harlow scolded the psychological profession for ignoring affection and bonding as an essential part of the childhood experience. "Love is a wondrous state, deep, tender, and rewarding," he said in his opening remarks. "But so far as love or affection is concerned, psychologists have failed in this mission."

Other investigators soon began to recognize and herald the bonding process. The famous child psychologist John Bowlby wrote about the place the mother-child bond plays in the proper health and development of humankind. "Bowlby made a case for the intimate link between mother and infant as a long-ago-evolved system, something we share with other sexually reproducing organism," writes Meredith F. Small in *Our Babies, Ourselves.*[17]

> The bond is elicited, he felt, by an innate urge in the mother to protect the infant, and when babies cry or fret, that response is stimulated. From Bowlby's point of view, the idea of imprinting is also involved,

---

*Harry F. Harlow was an American Psychologist who provided a new understanding of human behavior and development through studies of the social behavior of monkeys.

because new mothers are highly receptive to their infants in all the sensory channels, including sight, smell, hearing, and especially touch. In other words, Bowlby felt the mother-infant bond has been selected over generations as a pattern of behavior that has helped individuals successfully produce and pass on genes by attaching to and bringing up their infants.[18]

Referring to the bonding process as "attachment parenting" in their classic 1992 work *The Baby Book,* Dr. William Sears and Martha Sears, R.N., tell us bonding has been around "as long as there have been mothers and babies. It is, in fact, only recently that this style of parenting has needed a name at all, for it is basically the commonsense parenting we all would do if left to our own healthy resources."[19]

In a sidebar the Searses maintain that attachment-parented children, statistically speaking, enjoy better health than nonbonded children. The authors insist that the children are more sensitive, more intelligent, empathetic, easier to discipline, and tend to be attached to human beings rather than to physical things.*

Jean MacKeller, wife of a Western doctor practicing in Uganda, passed on a number of fascinating observations to Joseph Chilton Pearce concerning the extremely close relationship between Ugandan mothers and their infant babies, thereby showing us the connection between all lovingly bonded mothers and their children, wherever they resided.[20] According to MacKeller's account, Ugandan babies go diaper free, yet appear never to defecate or urinate on their mother's skin. How is this possible? MacKeller asked a Ugandan woman.

"Oh, we go to the bushes," the mother replied.

"How do you know it is time for the child to go to the bathroom at that exact moment?" MacKeller queried.

The mother was perplexed by the question, and had to think about

---

*The Sears' work in their many books has helped to spearhead a growing awareness of the importance of *attachment parenting*—another term for bonding—for children, their parents, their families, and all of society.

it. "Well," she finally replied, "How do you know when you have to go to the bathroom?"

A patient of mine who had just become a new mother once confided in me that she knew when her child needed to be breastfed several minutes before the child actually began to cry.

"How can you tell?" I asked her.

"I can hear it in my breasts," the woman answered.

Similarly, a friend once asked my wife, "How can you afford to spend so much time with your child?"

"How can I afford not to?" she replied.

Dalit's meaning is that the most valuable thing in the world is to be with your child, but many do not have a life situation that makes it possible to be at home full time. This does not mean that you are not a good parent. You also have to provide food and shelter for your family. When precious time is limited, you must remember to have real quality time. You must be completely focused on your child and not distracted by outside influences. Even if you have a very demanding career there are many creative ways to work and still practice conscious parenting. It is important that you communicate with your employer about alternatives to your regular work schedule. Many employers allow their employees to bring their baby to work with them. Some companies today provide areas for babies to play with supervision. Some employers may allow a new mother to work from home, or do so for two or three days a week. Or you could get permission to leave work for twenty minutes to go home to nurse your baby and return to work. If you work for a large or a small company, *ask your bosses:* you may be surprised. You may become the first to set a new level of concern for new mothers.

AN ALTERNATIVE BIRTH: CONTINUING THE STORY OF OUR CHILD'S ARRIVAL

As we told in chapter 1, Dalit and I became pregnant after moving to New York City. Here is a continuation of our odyssey.

Meet Your New M.D.

Dalit took an EPT home pregnancy test—in fact, she took two of them.

Her woman's instinct plus the glow generated from obvious physical changes that were already taking place in her body confirmed for her before the test results that a child was growing in her womb. As the tests showed, she was right.

We scheduled a formal interview with an obstetrician. The doctor we chose to oversee our pregnancy and to deliver our baby was a former colleague of mine and was—at least so I'd heard from several female patients of mine—an excellent gynecologist-obstetrician.

On the day of our first appointment we arrived at his office filled with anticipation. The nurse behind the glass window greeted us with a cool nod and was crisp in ordering us to take our seats and wait along with the other—we counted them—twenty-two pregnant women. The doctor, she cautioned, had a particularly busy schedule that day.

Her assessment was quite accurate. Our birthing mentor was not available for—we clocked it—two hours and seven minutes.

When our number finally came up, we were ushered into his large, empty, white office, and here we waited for another quarter of an hour.

Finally, the great man entered. He gave us a blank stare, nodded, and seated himself behind his desk without a word. We had been friendly at one time and had once chatted briefly on the phone about old times. He clearly knew who I was. Why was he playing the role of detached professional?

Our new doctor proceeded to administer a four-minute physical examination of my wife. Then he had his nurse perform a sonogram to make sure the pregnancy was, as he termed it, "valid."

After this, we went back to his office to ask a few questions about the hospital and the delivery. He informed us that we were putting the cart before the horse and that we would talk about hospital matters when we were closer to the date of birth. Anyway, he asserted, it would all be taken care of. We didn't have to worry.

After rummaging through his files looking for God knows what, the doctor sat down at his desk again, wrote silently and mysteriously for several minutes, looked up, gave us a forced smile, told us everything was in order health-wise, and said that he would see us back in his office next month. Dismissing us, he added, "Call if you have any questions."

Back in the waiting room, the nurse presented us with a bill for five hundred dollars—"Please pay before you leave."

As we walked out of the office onto the street, my wife and I looked at each other in dazed befuddlement. Over a cup of tea we asked ourselves: Where was the friendly support, the wise counsel, the at-home instructions, the preparatory teaching for what we both were hoping would be the most enriching experience we would ever undergo in all our lives as husband and wife: the birth of our child?

It was certainly not to be found in this doctor's office. We decided to bail out on this unforthcoming professional and retain the services of another obstetrician—one, we hoped, who was more helpful and had a better bedside manner.

I asked around among my doctor friends and finally settled on a woman obstetrician, who, I was assured, was as compassionate as she was knowledgeable. After all, she had delivered the babies of most of the doctors and their wives at her large New York City hospital.

Round Two and Round Three

This time, we sat in the waiting room for only forty-five minutes. We were still feeling ecstatic, flying with the joy of our pregnancy. The delay seemed inconsequential.

When we were finally seated before our new obstetrician, she chuckled a great deal in a pleasant way and gave my wife a physical examination that seemed longer and more thorough than the previous one—but she too deflected our questions and seemed almost annoyed when my wife asked what she could do to overcome the morning sickness that was giving her a world-class case of nausea every day.

The doctor was Indian by origin, thus I thought perhaps she would recommend a natural or Auyervedic remedy. But no, not at all. She shook her head with a peevish frown and told Dalit to take Tums.

This time the bill at the desk was for six hundred dollars.

Now my wife and I are persistent people, and both of us still entertained the hope that somewhere there was an obstetrician who was willing to provide us at least a modicum of emotional support and instructive information.

So once more, we went back into the fray. This time, though, we would go straight to the top. The following week I scheduled an appointment with the chief of staff in obstetrics at a major New York City hospital. This physician, we were told, had written one of the seminal books on fetal development. He was world famous as a media expert on child rearing and was a trailblazer in improved birthing techniques.

This time, instead of sitting for what seemed like a lifetime in a waiting room and then being marched into a sterile, white cubicle, we were ushered into a beautifully furnished apartment. The main room was paneled in mahogany. Hand-colored eighteenth-century Italian medical prints hung on the walls. The doctor himself was seated at a colossal Napoleonic desk. He smiled at us genially as we entered. No waiting room blues in this office. Behind him three computers hummed away.

Our first question to him was the same we had asked of both previous candidates: How could my wife control the morning sickness that continued to defy all conventional remedies?

The doctor furrowed his brow, shook his head, then turned and typed into one of his computers for several minutes. A moment later, five pages emerged from the printer, slid down a shoot, and shuffled themselves into a neat packet on his desk. He picked it up and handed it to me.

On this formidable read-out, in small, single-spaced print, was a list of what he informed us was every remedy currently known to medical science, both natural and conventional, for the treatment of nausea and morning sickness.

My wife and I perused the list for a minute and quickly found it overwhelming in length and complexity. I mentioned that it looked pretty complicated and asked which of the formulas he most recommended.

He smiled. "Whichever one works best for you."

For the next ten minutes of our fifteen-minute appointment our doctor then proceeded to tell us all about the new book he had just written on childbirth and how it was revolutionizing the "birth industry," as he put it.

As we rose to leave, he invited us to attend his book signing on the following Tuesday night on 23rd Street. Come at seven o'clock sharp, he said. There would be free coffee and punch, and each copy would be discounted 10 percent for professionals such as myself.

The bill in the waiting room was ready for us: $825.

Seek and Ye Shall Stumble On

We wondered: What do we do now?

The idea of placing ourselves into the mercenary, loveless hands of the medical professionals we had met so far was unthinkable. We both agreed: Bedside manner, proper instruction, and a genuinely supportive attitude were as important to successful childbirth as medical technique. At least, they were as important as medical technique for *our* childbirth—and all three were roundly missing from the members of the conventional doctor establishment we had interviewed so far.

Meanwhile, time was marching on. My wife's abdomen was growing larger by the day. What were our alternatives?

After many hours of discussion and after mentally reviewing much of Joe Pearce's work and the many reports I'd read through the years on natural childbirth, at the recommendation of a colleague whose wife had gone this route, we finally did something that until now our conditioned fears had vetoed: we made an appointment to speak with a midwife.

Though my wife and I were both well versed in natural healing modalities, neither of us knew much about midwifery. The subject was not spoken of in the popular press or even mentioned by most alternative or even naturopathic doctors. For all intents and purposes, it didn't exist at all. We had certainly never heard any mention of it in the obstetrician's office or in the obstetric medical journals and parenting magazines we pored over—and anyway, wasn't midwifery an anachronism, a residue of the bloodletting days of screaming childbirth on farmhouse floors and charity wards?

To find out more about this frankly nerve-wracking alternative, we did a bit of investigating before our appointment.

To our amazement we learned that midwifery is part of a large, organized, and growing grassroots birthing trend that is currently practiced in every state of the Union. I had known little of this movement before Dalit became pregnant even though a good deal of my work was focused on the field of alternative health care.

We also found out that midwives are not simply birth mechanics or towel-handlers at a delivery. They are skilled medical professionals. Before practicing their profession, they must earn a two-year master's degree in their field, then pass rigorous state testing, and then undergo a prolonged period of on-site learning and apprenticeship. Many start out as registered nurses who go on to earn a master's degree in midwifery. After meeting basic educational requirements, the midwife may take a certification exam administered by a major professional organization such as the North American Registry of Midwives. Most significantly, while most obstetricians are trained to look for pathology and have lost trust in a pregnant woman's natural ability to birth, midwives believe deeply that if proper conditions are created, any healthy pregnant woman can give birth with a minimum of help from other people and no need for medical intervention.

My wife and I were intrigued—so intrigued that at our first meeting we were not all that surprised to discover that our midwife-to-be was a veritable encyclopedia of obstetric knowledge and professional expertise. What did surprise and delight us was that she also understood how fragile and elemental an event childbearing is for a pregnant couple and how essential it is that those who oversee the blessed event stand beside the parents with compassionate advocacy and support.

This imposing woman, we further learned from testimonials, had already delivered more than two hundred babies—all of them safely and soundly—and seemed to know everything there was to know on the subject of childbirth. Nor was her knowledge limited to the delivery process alone. It encompassed a spectrum of related subjects, including nutrition, natural pain control, postpartum bonding methods, useful medications, body massage, pre- and post-natal exercises, psychological self-care, and many other tricks of the birthing trade that women who go the conventional medical route are almost never told.

Clearly, we had found what we were looking for.

Making a Birth Plan

Each subsequent visit we made to our midwife lasted for at least an hour. During these sessions our questions were answered in full, and a great deal of additional information—some of it unanticipated and unexpected—was deposited in our ever-enlarging knowledge bank.

Then one day during a teaching session, our midwife informed us that it was time to write out a birth plan—that is, to devise a document describing in detail the ways in which we wanted our child to be born. She told us that it should include the location of the birth (hospital, birthing center, or at home); religious ceremonies to be practiced; the father's role in delivery; instructions about cutting the umbilical cord; and actions and activities to avoid. Whatever personal preferences both Dalit and I had should be listed on the plan. Our midwife promised us that these instructions would be followed to every extent possible on the day of the birth.

Yet, though my wife and I were deeply impressed by everything we had seen and heard so far in this brave new world of natural birthing, we entertained fears about delivering a child at home. We asked ourselves the questions parents-to-be often ask: Isn't natural birth risky? What if something goes wrong, medically speaking? What if Dalit hemorrhages or the baby becomes lodged in the birth canal and there is no time to get to the hospital?

As we later learned, these fears can be handled fully and addressed by any practiced midwife. Nonetheless, in our case inbred hesitations carried the day: On our birth plan we indicated that we were unsure about home birth. What were our other options?

Our midwife understood these reservations immediately. She suggested that we compromise and that our child be delivered at one of the natural birthing centers that had recently opened in several New York City hospitals. This way, she explained, our child could be brought into the world by the two of us in an attractive birthing chamber with whomever we choose in attendance. In case anything went wrong medically, hospital attention would be a single flight up.

This idea fully accommodated our concerns. We began visiting hospitals in the city and soon chose Roosevelt Hospital in Manhattan. It ran a beautifully appointed and well-equipped birthing center. Roosevelt's special natural unit was separate from the rest of the hospital but was just a flight of stairs down from the maternity ward. The delivery room itself, designed to resemble a sleek studio apartment, was furnished with comfortable chairs, Oriental carpets, mahogany tables, a large Jacuzzi bath, and a queen-sized birthing bed that was not unlike our own bed at home. Attached to the apartment was a small room to accommodate friends and family who wished to attend the birth.

We had found what we were looking for down to the smallest detail. Now we simply had to wait.

The Most Common Mistake

One of the most sage pieces of advice our midwife passed on to us during our instructional sessions was that on the eve of giving birth, pregnant women in our society tend to panic and go to the hospital too soon. The panic trigger, she warned, is pulled prematurely the moment contractions begin.

Because they are not tutored by their physicians in the mechanics of contractions and how they really work, mothers-to-be overreact at the first tightening sensations, not knowing that these prebirthing cramps can sometimes go on for several days without bearing fruit.

Jittery and uncertain, mothers then rush to the hospital before they are ready to give birth. Once there, they either are told they are experiencing false labor and sent home after a grueling day's wait or are forced to sit hour after hour in an anxiety-provoking hospital room while they dilate, which at times concludes with labor being artificially induced. This, in turn, can cause painful, tumultuous labor, decreased uterine blood flow, and reduction of oxygen to the baby, among a host of other side effects (much more on this later).

To avoid a premature trip to the delivery room, we waited until Dalit was absolutely certain that she was ready. One day—it was a holiday—she was busy making a meal and polishing silver. Then her water broke, and off we went.

The Day of Joy

The birthing room at Roosevelt Hospital was ready when we arrived. Our midwife, Anna, was waiting for us with several aides who would attend the birth, as was Sigrid Nelsson-Ryan, chief birth educator at Roosevelt Hospital. Our helpers began by filling the room with the aromatic candles we had requested in our birth plan and by playing a variety of classical music that we brought with us from home. Dalit's mother was there to watch and help.

From our formal lessons in birth education, we already knew what were integral needs for every delivering mother: the need for quiet and protected privacy, a sense of free choice concerning birthing postures (standing, sitting, walking, squatting), freedom to make sounds and perform physical gyrations and gestures. After all, the mother is now entering a condition of altered consciousness where intellectual activity is low and emotional and sensual awareness are working at full volume, just as nature intended. Any interruption of this altered awareness—such as a loud noise, bright lights, even an innocent question—forces the mother into the thinking part of her brain, where fear and doubt intrude and disturb dramatically the trancelike state necessary for a fully focused birth.

We therefore made sure that the birthing chamber was quiet and dimly lit; that Dalit could be alone if she wished or with her mother and me if she wished; that she had the option to move around the room, remain sedentary, or lie down. Her needs were first on the list; her wishes were our commands.

As Dr. Michel Odent writes:

> To meet the mammalian needs means first to satisfy the need for privacy, since all mammals have a strategy not to feel observed when giving birth. It also means satisfying the need to feel secure: the female of a mammal in the jungle cannot give birth as long as there is a predator around. It is significant that when a laboring woman has complete privacy and feels secure, she often finds herself in typically mammalian postures, for example, on all fours.[21]

Dalit slipped into the Jacuzzi, where for the next six hours she continued to dilate slowly under the warm, swirling water. The pulsing jets eased her entire body and reduced the pain of the contractions, also relaxing our child in utero. At the same time, the warm water helped the groin and abdominal muscles loosen and become flexible, preparing her for the intense pushing activity that would soon follow. Many studies have shown that fretful mothers experience a more difficult and painful delivery than women who are calm and centered. All those in attendance that day did everything in their power to ensure that Dalit was comfortable and anxiety free.

As the hours went by, the contractions built steadily, each one lasting approximately a minute. As they became more frequent and intense,

I did what I'd been taught to do in our training sessions. I coached my wife, holding my stopwatch, speaking to her in loving tones, talking her from beginning to end of the rising and falling spasms, each time using an image we had both chosen: the metaphoric depiction of waves washing in and breaking on the shore. Because our subconscious mind thinks in images, this primal view spoke directly to her body-mind at the deepest level.

"Here comes the next wave," I said, as the contraction arrived. "Now we're fifteen seconds into it. Hold on, here it comes, rolling in from the ocean . . . thirty seconds . . . it's reaching its crest, we're already halfway through, hold on . . . forty-five seconds, it's crested now, almost at the end. . . . Now it's sixty seconds, the wave has passed—we made it!"

Then she relaxed in the swirling water and was pain free for several minutes until the next wave arrived. When the pain did come, Dalit reacted to it in whatever way seemed most appropriate: by groaning, laughing, howling. "The key for rediscovering the universal needs of women in labor," writes Odent regarding a woman's varied reactions to delivery, "is to interpret a phenomenon which is well-known to certain mothers and midwives who have experience of undisturbed birth. It is the fact that when a woman is giving birth by herself, without any medication, there is a time when she has an obvious tendency to cut herself off from the world, as if going to another planet. (In a book called *Storey's Guide to Raising Meat Goats,* I learned that during the first parts of labor, goats gaze off into the faraway distance and are quite unreachable.) She dares to do what she would never dare to do in her daily social life; for example scream or swear. She can find herself in the most unexpected postures, making the most unexpected noises. This means that she is reducing the control by the neocortex in her brain [the thinking part of the mind]. *This reduction of neocortical activity is the most important aspect of birth physiology from a practical point of view.*"[22]

Dalit continued this uninhibited letting-go for some time until her contractions began to come in rapid, regular succession. Finally, she felt the pressure of the baby's head pushing through the birth canal and crowning. At this moment, she climbed out of the tub, and aided by the midwife and attendants, she settled herself into the birthing bed.

Here, in a minimum of pain and in a serene, candle-lit room with celestial music playing, surrounded by her loving husband, her mother, and friendly faces in an atmosphere of ineffable joy, within ten minutes the midwife and Sigrid had helped my wife bring our uncrying infant into this wide, bright world.

Who among us would not wish to be born in such a way?

A Taste of the New Parenting

As our birth plan stated, I stood by Dalit's side and held our new son in my hands as he emerged. I hugged his tiny, wet body to my chest in an epiphany of gratitude, amazement, and love. Then I placed him on my wife's stomach and watched in a kind of ecstasy as instinctively he crawled his way up to the area of Dalit's heart and placed his head over her left breast.

Having been taught in advance about the "crawl reflex" that impels newborns to inch their way by themselves up to the breast, my wife was fully prepared. She guided our child's mouth to her nipple, and he began to drink peacefully with his umbilical cord still attached.

After ten minutes, when the cord stopped throbbing and the baby was breathing freely on his own, I cut the cord myself, then picked him up and hugged him again, gazing steadily into his eyes. (Despite the old wives' tale that newborns have no vision, they are actually programmed to see at a distance of ten to twelve inches the moment they are born, a process that helps them bond with their new parents.) I then handed him to my wife's mother, who made similar eye contact, and she then returned him to Dalit.

Dalit, in turn, followed her natural impulse to knead and rub the child's body gently from head to foot. We had been taught that when first born, children are covered with a shiny mucus coating called *vernix* that protects their tender skin and keeps them warm. In ordinary hospital delivery rooms babies are washed immediately after birth, then bundled up in linens that provide a synthetic substitute for maternal warmth. In the process, this precious coating is rinsed off their bodies entirely and is lost forever. In older, wiser cultures, this coating is always left intact, which allows the mother to massage it into the child's skin so that it can provide all the benefits nature intended, some of which are not yet fully known.

That night, my wife and I slept together with our new son next to us in the large birthing-room bed. The following morning we returned home, jubilant, relaxed, and anxious to begin the journey of child raising that awaited us. We had just experienced a taste, the first round, the first step of the new parenting.

FIXING THE WORLD

For several weeks after Kesem's birth, I found myself bothered by the realization that many mothers and fathers in our society have been systematically deprived of the experience in which we had just gloried. I wondered: How many parents have been denied the partnered joy of a free-from-fear childbirth and the elated bonding moments that follow?

How many of our fathers have sat anxiously in a sterile hospital waiting room, leafing through magazines, staring unseeingly at the TV overhead, not allowed to participate in the most awesome event that is likely to grace their lives? How many of our mothers have lain in hospital beds in a narcotic stupor, surrounded by aloof strangers, half-aware and half-terrified as medical technicians pull from the womb their baby, who is as fully numbed and frightened as its mother?

As for myself, even after the blissful delivery of our child, it took a number of conversations with health care professionals who were friendly to the ideas of new parenting, plus another year of research, for me to understand fully the important lessons I had learned from my study and from my experience of Kesem's birth.

First, it was apparent to me that so many of the traditional methods for organic birthing and heart-to-heart child rearing, which societies everywhere (including our own) had embraced for so many centuries, have been swept away by modern medicine.

Second, in the process of destroying the old ways, the medicalization of a woman's childbearing functions and the giving over of all delivery-room power to doctors and machines has reduced the once radiantly blissful moment of birth to the status of an emergency-room operation.

Third, the separation of the mother from the child at birth, which denies the child essential bonding, is emblematic of many more mother-child separations to come, culminating finally in institutions such as daycare and in a society that does not like its children very much and does not really want them around a great deal of the time. I compared this to the many child-friendly societies of the world in which children are invariably kept close to home in the early years of life. There, family, friends, neighbors, and even strangers dote on them and just about everyone in the culture looks on them with admiration, respect, delight, and love. (In a number of cultures, infants are doted on, but children are often seen as individuals who can bring in money to the family. In disadvantaged homes in many parts of India, for example, children are expected to work and earn much sooner than in this country—and in many parts of the world, children perform work that is hard and dangerous. Poverty is poverty, no matter where it occurs, and an infant who suckles at the breast soon turns into a child who requires food and clothing. This is the reality of the poor. We can't idealize this experience. An infant is not always welcomed—especially when there is sickness and poverty and caring for it soon becomes downright hard.) For the sake of our children and the children of the world, we teach and model compassion and charity to our child for an awareness of the poor and hungry. In our home we have a charity box to which we all contribute regularly. We also pray together as a family that world hunger and poverty will end soon in our days.

Last, and perhaps most terrifying, the more I looked into the effects of techno-based childbirth and the lack of child-parent bonding that follows, the more I realized that many of the most severe woes our society faces today are linked to the ways in which our culture births, raises, and educates its children. The medicalized model of child raising makes a major contribution to the disintegration of our health and safety as a nation, to our mental well-being, to our national character, and to our highest, finest dreams.

All these notions considered, throughout the chapters that follow, I will play the part of bell ringer and one who warns, telling you many things you may not wish to hear. I will also give you information that flies in the face of our culture's most cherished assumptions concerning childbirth and child rearing.

I am sorry about this, but not really—for if you heed the remarkable body of information I will pass along to you and take time to test it out in your own life, this effort will pay off a thousand-fold, for yourself and, even more, for your child. At the least, it will ensure that your young one is brought up to be a healthier, happier, better-adjusted person than he or she might have been if this remarkable new body of child-raising knowledge had not come your way. The new parenting can be that powerful and that important a force in a family's life. There are those people who, for whatever reason, could not avail themselves of a birth experience like ours. It is important to add: Even if folks experience a birth that isn't natural and organic, it's not too late to begin the process of bonding.

Once you discover these new options, moreover—once you discover the hard scientific evidence that has been kept from you until now, once you learn of the remarkably toxic and injurious methods of childbirth and raising children that have become the norm in our culture and that are in your power to avoid, once you discover the safe and healthy alternatives to these methods—perhaps you will not only wish to put them into practice but also will want to tell the parents in the world that there is another way, a better way.

As this word spreads, modern civilization will find itself shifting away from the darkness and toward the light. Why? Because if we follow the tenets of the new parenting, we are also, as a matter of course, applying an ancient healing principle that Jewish sages refer to as *tik-kun*. Translated from the Hebrew, this word means "to rectify" or "to fix." In its most common use, it refers to righting wrongs, to making things better for everyone; to repairing our own life and, by so doing, helping to repair the life of the world—for these two parts of the whole, ourselves and the world, are ever linked.

In the process of applying tikkun, what's more, the boys and girls and men and women reared in our culture benefit in ways we can scarcely imagine and become less prone to the social and psychological ills that are so endemic in modern society.

EVERYONE PROSPERS

This opinion is not just my own. Currently, there is a grassroots trend among parents—estimated to be ten million strong—that follows many of the ideas that are seminal to the new parenting. These same ideas are likewise embraced by a large number of doctors, psychologists, and researchers, many of whom have written extensively on the subject and many of whom we will meet in the chapters that follow.

These far-seeing men and women believe, as I do, that every teacher and guardian, every doctor and nurse, every parent and grandparent, every aunt and uncle, every stepparent and godparent and parent-to-be—anyone, in fact, who cares about children and who wishes to make a better world—should be informed of new parenting ideas. This body of knowledge, they insist, should be communicated from person-to-person, from country-to-country, and it can't wait for tomorrow or the day after tomorrow. It should be communicated now, this very moment.

This world-fixing model may be tall order, but isn't it time? Indeed, isn't time running out?

⁓

The great Persian poet Jalal al-Din Rumi ends many of his narrative tales with the resonant phrase: "This story hath no end." Rumi is right, of course, because he is referring to the story of life, love, death, and rebirth, which indeed has no end.

Our story, on the other hand, the story of birth, child raising, and the sacred parental bond, is not about endings. It is about beginnings. As T. S. Eliot writes in one of his four quartets, ". . . my end is my beginning."

What this means from the standpoint of the new parenting is that as parents and families, we can all embark on a journey that concludes when the butterfly child we have nurtured, in the best ways we know how, finally bursts forth from the cocoon of childhood and flies abroad into the world with strength, serenity, vigor, an infinite capacity to learn, and an eye upon a star. Once this process takes place we can rest on our laurels—but then we also begin to make a strange and marvelous discovery: By practicing new parenting techniques, transformative things happen to parents as well as to their offspring. What's more, by attending consciously to a child's true inner needs, you, as a parent, can perhaps amend some of the deeper damage that was done to you as a young person by your own parents. By means of some inscrutable wonderworking along the silent way, through some mysterious psychological alchemy, when we raise a child who is adjusted and whole, we repair our own past in the process.

Yet how, through this process of child rearing, can we restore the wounded, deprived parts of our childhood that seem so irrevocably past and broken? It is true: As you practice the fine art of parental bonding, as your child matures, and as time passes, you begin gradually to earn a special taste, a unique and unmistakable sensation that something ancient and aching is being healed within you. Exactly how this process works and why it works at all is a mystery we shall explore further in this book.

There is a saying heard from time to time in the mental health profession: It is never too late to have a happy childhood. The truth is, it is never too late to mend or rekindle the inner child. The energies and delights that we imagined to be extinguished inside us long ago when we were too young and helpless to know what was being done to us can be reawakened and set right. It is never too late, as the Hindus say, to be "twice born." In the process, as we heal ourselves and take back portions of our lost childhood, we also have the pleasure of bestowing the gift of physical, emotional, and mental health on another human being—on our beloved son or daughter—to give our child a childhood devoid of fear and blame, then watch as the positive results flow over into our family life, our social life, our community, and ultimately the world around us.

Each of the following chapters profiles a different stage and different set of needs in the early life of a child. Each provides the type of factual information you will need to begin, but are not likely to find, in a majority of other books on the subject.

As Joseph Chilton Pearce writes:

Our children have been signaling us for years that things are critically wrong for them. In our anxiety-ridden concern to "equip them fully for life" we have been deaf and blind to their distress calls. Perhaps at this critical point for the survival of the species, we can do more than make another futile gesture toward patching up the holes in our exhausted system of ideas. Perhaps we can seize this cubic centimeter of chance that history is giving us and move, not just to correct some of the more blatant and tragic errors we have made with children, but to actually turn again to that three-billion-year development lying within us, that uncanny wisdom of the body clearly programmed into the child as unbending intent. In learning to live again, we can learn of this wisdom and allow our children (and so ourselves) to become the free, whole individuals this good earth has prepared us to be.[23]

Onward and upward.

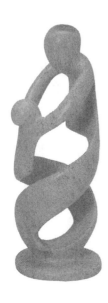

3

A Child's First Schoolhouse

Learning in the Womb

How we influence our kids can make superstars out of them with consciousness. Without consciousness we are probably doomed.

DR. BRUCE LIPTON, *NATURE, NURTURE AND THE POWER OF LOVE: THE BIOLOGY OF CONSCIOUS PARENTING*

THERE IS A MUCH-QUOTED saying among fathers and mothers who practice natural child rearing: The education of your child begins the moment your child is born. The first day, the first hour, the first instant of life outside the mother's uterus and your little one begins absorbing information at a rate approaching warp speed. Learning is as natural to a newborn (neonate) as breathing.

At the same time, due to an abundance of scientific data that has appeared in the past thirty to forty years, and thanks to the work and dedication of new parenting medical professionals around the world, it has now become increasingly clear that human education starts a good deal sooner than the moment of birth. It begins, we now know, in utero—in the womb. Here, it flourishes even in the early days following conception. It then picks up momentum as the child grows, reaching a crescendo of cognitive and sensory development in the last trimester of pregnancy.

What is learned during this preciously critical period lodges firmly in the very depths of a child's being. It remains there from birth to death, as deeply imprinted upon the heart and mind as a fiery brand.

PRESENT AT THE CREATION

Even during the first and second trimester of pregnancy, an unborn child—the prenate—starts receiving and assimilating relatively complex sensory and emotional information. Cognitive and perceptual learning, along with the underpinnings of personality and ego formation, all progress to surprising and hitherto unsuspected levels of development. Many prenatal studies indicate that a fetus of six or seven months is capable of reasoning, if in a primitive way. Observations also demonstrate that in-womb memories function on a relatively sophisticated level.

There are many other forms of prenate learning as well. During pregnancy, for example, a mother's slumber routines exert a profound influence on the type of sleep patterns her unborn child will one day experience and on the moods and temperament her child will display as an adult. There is even evidence that a pregnant mother's dreams may affect the quality and length of the prenate's birth.

Of equal importance, as we shall see, is the fact that a child's in-womb senses, once thought to be quasi-dormant for all three trimesters of pregnancy, are capable of hearing, seeing, and touching to a far greater degree than was ever supposed, and that unborn children are adept at tuning into activities both inside and outside their mother's bodies, forming lasting impressions from the messages they receive.

Spectacularly significant is the recent discovery that in-womb learning is not simply a preprogrammed biological event that unfolds according to the ironclad commands of a child's DNA. Genes governing health, emotions, and brainpower can also be controlled—and even changed—by the impressions a fetus receives from the outside world. Indeed, the more we learn about life in the womb, the more we learn that the genetic code is highly alterable by the degree of nurturance an unborn child receives.

The nature of these environmental impressions, as we learn from the remarkable work of biologist Dr. Bruce Lipton and others, depends to a large extent on the ways in which parents care for their in-womb child and, of almost equal importance, the ways in which they relate to one another during the course of pregnancy. Even more astonishing, there is strong scientific evidence to suggest that genetic markers are affected and altered by parents' physical health and mental attitudes before the male sperm and female ovum actually unite—that is, before the act of fertilization takes place. Further, these parental behavior patterns can affect personality formation in the child-to-be as many as sixty days prior to conception.

Finally, we now understand that the prenate's ability to experience mood, arousal, and response to stimuli are programmed into its developing neurons and that the mother's emotional disposition during pregnancy affects a child's mental and physical health significantly. During pregnancy, a cascade of hormones and neurotransmitters flow from the mother into the fetus, sending subtle but notable messages to the developing child and, in the process, "firing" these neurons in ways previous generations of scientists never thought possible. If the neurons are fired in a positive way, a healthy child results; if they are turned on in a negative way, trouble looms.

Certainly such concepts give new meaning to the new parenting dictum that it is never too early to begin teaching your child.

BUT FREUD DISAGREES

Through the centuries a select number of parents have understood intuitively the importance of providing loving and on-going communication with their in-womb child. In addition, for many years a small group of scientists knew the secrets of in-womb parenting. During the early Renaissance, for example, Leonardo da Vinci noted that the formation of a child's knowledge base starts almost immediately after its moment of conception. He recognized the critical relationship between the mother's behavior and the child's in-utero development. "The things desired by the mother," he wrote, "are often impressed on the child [in the womb]."[1]

Leonardo's famous remark, *Ogni nostra cognizioni principia dai sentimenti* (there is nothing in the intellect which was not first in the senses), is a telling and profound observation of prenatal learning and one whose application will become increasingly apparent in the pages that follow. Unborn children, many have understood, enjoy a rich, busy life even before they are born.

But Freud and his colleagues did not agree. According to early theories of psychoanalysis and of early to mid-twentieth century psychiatric thinking (based, it should be said, on far less scientific research than is available today), a child's personality does not begin to develop until the second to third year of life. True learning, early psychiatrists maintained, goes hand-in-hand with ego formation, which does not shift into high gear until a child walks and talks. Before this time, their thinking was that children are scarcely more than passive packages of instincts and reflexes. These packages generate no real thoughts and emotions, as we understand them. Instead, the child operates in a purely reactive state of consciousness, caring only for the satisfaction of primal needs— movement, rest, food, sensation, attention, and security—a state akin to, as Shakespeare describes it, "a drowsy after-dinner sleep."[2]

◠

Though most turn-of-the century psychiatrists adopted Freud's point of view, occasional dissenting opinions were heard. In his 1924 book, *The Trauma of Birth*, Dr. Otto Rank recognized that the origins of neurotic development can often be traced back to painful and frightening sensations that bedevil a child at the moment of delivery. Rank, a disciple of Freud, insisted that adult neurotic and even psychotic disorders displayed on the psychiatrist's couch cannot be understood fully without first helping patients to come to terms with the shock of their own birth.

In the 1950s, the Hungarian psychoanalyst Nandor Fodor insisted that every high-anxiety dream we suffer is somehow related to memories of emerging from our mother's womb. Francis Mott, a disciple of Fodor's, went so far as to develop a psychology based entirely on the natal experience, focusing on analysis of birth trauma, the dreams of patients in adulthood, and the role played by birth and birth trauma in traditional mythologies around the world.

Yet despite parental intuition, plus an occasional voice raised in the scientific wilderness, for the first half of the twentieth century, medical researchers gave short shrift to the study of in-womb psychology. In the process they failed to recognize gestation as a critical phase in personality development and simultaneously ignored overwhelming evidence that an unborn child possesses a boundless capacity to think, feel, and perceive—and thus to learn.

FOUR WAYS YOUR BABY LEARNS BEFORE BIRTH

Today, scientists of new parenting have progressed far beyond the classic theory of the comatose fetus, demonstrating in clinical as well as theoretical ways that an unborn child's learning potential encompasses far more than passive reflex and automaton-like reactivity. Sensory learning, sleep patterns, memory, and even tendencies toward peacefulness or violence are established to some degree before a child is born.

Let's look more closely at these four prenate learning encounters:

1. Sleep patterns
2. Memory and reasoning
3. The five senses
4. Mental health

Sleep Patterns

Our lifelong sleep and mood patterns are determined to a marked degree by our experience in the womb. In their groundbreaking book, *The Secret Life of the Unborn Child,* Thomas Verney and John Kelly report in-womb sleep studies carried out by the Swiss pediatrician Dr. R. Stirnimann.[3] According to Dr. Stirnimann's findings, an individual's lifetime sleep routines are firmly established in utero by the nocturnal practices of the mother.

To prove his point, Dr. Stirnimann selected two groups of pregnant women: One group had a marked tendency to rise early in the morning; the other preferred to sleep late. When the children of these mothers were born, Stirnimann studied their routines. According to his findings, the mothers who were out of bed at the crack of dawn produced early-waking babies—who remained early-wakers into their grownup years. At the same time, late-sleeping mothers produced late-sleeping infants—and, true to form, these children grew up to become late-sleeping adults.

Supplementary to Stirnimann's findings, it is now fairly well established from a number of laboratory studies that mothers who have frequent nightmares during pregnancy tend to have shorter and easier birth deliveries than mothers who do not remember their dreams. Such nocturnal frights are one of nature's ingenious ways of helping mothers process their pregnancy-related worries and cope with the states of apprehension and dread. In the process, the mother's anxiety levels are lowered, and the prenate's anxiety levels drop accordingly. Anxiety-ridden dreams, in fact, appear to help mothers arrive at resolutions to conflicts and fears that they are normally incapable of solving with their conscious minds. In sum, bad dreams—and perhaps good dreams in certain circumstances—purify much of the negative mental material that accumulates in a pregnant mother's unconscious, helping her to remain buoyant and, as a kind of reflex, producing a more optimistic child as well.

In a complimentary way, animal studies indicate that high stress levels in a mother rat can produce profound behavioral, sleep, and endocrine abnormalities in her adult offspring. These abnormalities mimic those found in depressed human patients, indicating that the prenatally stressed laboratory rat may serve as an indicator for depression and sleep abnormalities in human beings. For example, in a 1999 study in Belgium,[4] pregnant rats were subjected repeatedly to physical and environmental stressors. Along with rats used as controls, the prenatally stressed male offspring were then tested. Results showed that rats stressed in the womb displayed more disturbed sleep patterns than control rats and a decreased ability to adapt to abrupt shifts in the light-dark cycle. "Taken together," the researchers conclude, "our data indicate . . . that sleep disturbances in prenatally stressed rats are similar to those found in depressed patients support the usefulness of prenatal stress as a new animal model of depression."[5]

What about babies themselves? Do they experience sleep in a way that is comparable to adults, complete with dreams and REM (Rapid Eye Movement) periods? In his essay, "Some Aspects of Prenatal Parenting," Thomas Verney answers this question in a definitive way: "Recordings of the baby's brain waves at the beginning of the last trimester demonstrate that during sleep the baby exhibits REM (Rapid Eye Movement) motions. In adults REM sleep is almost always associated with dreaming. It follows, therefore, that babies must be dreaming by the seventh month."[6]

In order to generate a stream of associative mental impressions—even basic ones—the human brain must contain a stockpile of established memories to draw upon (thus showing proof of fetal recall) as well as a scrapbook of thoughts and images that compose the contents of the dream itself. The existence of REM sleep in prenates also demonstrates that children's unconscious minds are forming in-womb, and that they are beginning, however primitively, the cutting, sorting, and pasting together of an individual personality and worldview.

Finally, some scientists are coming to believe that a mother's dreams during pregnancy occasionally serve as a kind of extrasensory liaison between mother and child. Though this idea sounds far-fetched, this phenomenon has received a good deal of serious academic attention in the past several years. Varney and Kelly write,

> At Duke University, a special extrasensory research unit has been studying dreams for several decades. The American Association for the Advancement of Science, one of the most august and respected scientific bodies in the world, has been sufficiently impressed with the potential importance of extraordinary forms of communication to sponsor several research projects. It will be interesting to see what sort of results they eventually come up with.[7]

Memory and Reasoning

A prenate's memory and powers of reasoning are a good deal more developed than we supposed previously. Like the motion of our arms and legs, memory is a function that we take for granted and that we assume will always be with us, waiting to be put to use.

Yet like every human behavior, the ability to remember must be learned. Without the faculty of long-term and short-term recall we are unable to store and retain information. Without memory, we are unequipped to identify the faces of our friends and enemies alike. We forget how to put on a hat or slice our meat or turn off the water faucet. We are incapable of reading or writing and sometimes, as in advanced cases of Alzheimer's disease, of speaking. All such rote behaviors must first be learned, then stored away permanently for future reference in that mysterious vault in our mind.

For years, child health professionals had assumed that memory does not become operative until children develop speech and reason. Once again, the early-to-mid-twentieth-century notion of the mindless infant set the norm. Then, gradually, late-twentieth-century scientists began to question this assumption. "Whether fetal memory exists has attracted interest for many thousands of years," writes P. G. Hepper in a 1996 study on prenatal memory. "Evidence from fetal learning paradigms of classical conditioning, habituation, and exposure learning reveals that the fetus *does have a memory,*" says Hepper.[8]

Hepper goes on to describe a number of laboratory studies, all demonstrating the development and capacity of prenate memory. In one of these studies, published in the prestigious medical journal *Lancet,* pregnant mothers listened to a theme song from the children's TV show *Neighbors.* In one variation on the experiment, newborns stopped moving whenever they heard the *Neighbors* theme song and their heart rate relaxed into slower rhythms. When different theme melodies were played, the infants showed no reaction.[9]

In another variation of the study, ultrasound technology was used to observe prenates' reactions to the *Neighbors* theme. At thirty weeks of gestation, prenates showed no response or movement of any kind when the music was played. At thirty-seven weeks of gestation, however, the same prenates demonstrated a significant increase in movement and reactivity whenever they heard the tune. Prenates who were never exposed to the *Neighbors* theme at any point in their development showed no response at either age.

Conclusion? The ability to remember familiar stimuli is not merely a measurable faculty among the unborn; we can date its onset and development specifically to between thirty and thirty-seven weeks of gestation.[10]

When Dalit was pregnant, she and I spent some time singing to our unborn son a melody we had composed. Approximately two years after he was born we began singing the same song to him. This time, however, he put his hands over his ears and, becoming tearful, begged us to stop singing this particular song.

"Why?" we asked.

He replied: "Because it's too sad. Because it makes me cry."

Dalit and I theorized here that our son was recalling an earlier prenatal stage during which he was flooded with emotion.

Another interesting aspect of prebirth memory concerns the concept of *habituation.* This familiar psychological response can be defined formally as a lowered threshold of sensitivity to a specific stimuli or activity due to the constant repetition of that stimuli or activity. The first time you listen to a spine-tingling march or a dreamy love song, for example, you respond with arousal and delight. When it is played for the hundredth time, you scarcely hear it. Habituation has set in.

Transferring this script to the laboratory, studies show that a fetus develops habituation to external stimuli in much the same way as an adult. Prenates at thirty-six weeks, for instance, habituate gradually to the played sound of a 250 Hz tone—that is, at first they respond to this tone with movement and increased heartbeat, but on hearing the tone played dozens of times, their reaction level dips accordingly, just as yours or mine would. In laboratory studies, habituation to the sound of the mother's heartbeat has likewise been shown to take place among prenates.[11]

In short, like adults, unborn children can remember, become accustomed to, and perhaps even grow bored with repeated external impressions. This is all very human and even "mature."

Still another point to note concerning the capacity of fetal memory is the prenate's aptitude to recognize and prefer its own mother's voice. This ability does not simply bear witness to the unborn child's growing interest in the world around it. It may also be a survival mechanism, ensuring that the prenate recognizes his or her mother at the moment of birth and that the necessary attachment and bonding behavior follows this recognition.

One interesting study in this regard was carried out by Anthony DeCasper, professor of psychology at the University of North Carolina. Under DeCasper's watchful eye, pregnant mothers were instructed to read to their unborn infants from selected passages of Dr. Seuss's *The Cat in the Hat*. Several weeks after birth, each of these children was then exposed to a selection of different recordings, and each child could choose a favorite recording by modulating the degree of his or her sucking on a faux nipple. One of the selections included the voice of the child's mother reading *The Cat in the Hat* passages. After a few trials, almost all the newborns sucked at the false nipple at the speed necessary to hear their mother's voice.

In another experiment, this time carried out in France, mothers read a children's rhyme to their in utero child every day from week thirty-three of gestation to week thirty-seven. At the end of this time, though still in the womb, prenates signaled a distinct learning preference for the familiar poem rather than similar poems that were read to them.

Some children spontaneously recall birth events (even secrets) but expression of these memories is delayed until they can speak. Before they use words they can express their memories nonverbally by drawing pictures, acting out scenes using pantomime, pointing to the body locations, and by providing authentic sound effects for equipment (like suction devices) used at the birth. These children warn us that early memory and learning are real.[12]

The Five Senses

During the entire period of pregnancy, your child's five senses are functioning, often in remarkably sophisticated ways.

The sense of hearing. The ability to discern and respond to audio stimulation is the most measurable of the neonate's developing senses. According to the studies of Dr. Henry Truby, professor of pediatrics, linguistics, and anthropology at the University of Miami,[13] an in-utero child hears the sounds outside its mother's belly quite distinctly and moves in rhythm to them. If strident or angry words are shouted, Truby tells us, if the sounds of jackhammers and slamming doors fill the air, the child wiggles in an agitated way. If gentle sounds predominate, the child merges into a slow-motion dance that undulates in sync with what it hears.

The longer an in-utero child is exposed to unpleasant clamor or outcry, the more anxious and agitated it becomes. This anxiety eventually reaches a critical mass, lingering after the sounds themselves have ceased and continuing by the force of momentum alone—and in the process triggering negative chemical changes in the prenate's metabolism.

As far back as the 1940s, J. Bernard and L. Sontag observed that children move in set rhythms to their mother's speech.[14] In 1970 Brody and Axelrod advanced this discovery a notch, showing that in-womb movements are never random or accidental, but instead are always keyed to the voices and sounds the prenate hears from outside. Every movement, Brody and Axelrod found, has a definable meaning keyed to a prenate's mental and emotional mood.[15]

Four years later, at Boston University, William F. Condon and Louis Sander, using computers and high-speed film, went a step further, discovering that each child has a specific and unique repertoire of movements that are locked in perfect sync with the mother's speech patterns.[16] For example, every time a *kh* sound is uttered (as in *car* or *cap*), a child moves his head slightly to the left. Whenever an *rh* sound is made, the child may raise his or her right arm or may wiggle a pinky.

According to Joseph Chilton Pearce, Condon and Sander determined that it is possible to computerize an infant's total repertoire of movements in response to sound. The researchers started by making an artificial sound tape of speech parts, then they fed these sounds into the computer, matching the tape input to the infant's gyrations. "The computer would then predict the precise movements the infant would make to each of the sounds as they played," writes Pearce. "Condon and Sander would then play the tape to the infant, making [the child's] high-speed moves as they did so. They then checked the results frame by frame; invariably, each sound produced the matching physical movement as computerized and catalogued."[17]

Most remarkably, years later, when their one-time test subjects were adolescents and adults, Condon and Sander applied these findings to them. To their astonishment, they discovered that the subjects' reactions to these sounds were exactly the same as they were previously and that these reactions were now part of the subjects' permanent motor-system responses, which could be measured only on a micro level, and then only by sophisticated computer equipment. Yet there they were: a slightly turned head at the pronouncement of a *kh* sound or a microscopically wiggled pinky in response to an *rh*. The fundamentals of spoken language, it was apparent from this study, are already being learned and memorized in the mysterious cave of the womb.

Unborn children not only form habitual responses to spoken language. A child at five months of age enjoys a fully developed sense of hearing, and is capable of discerning and identifying a sophisticated range of sounds. According to Verney and Kelly, a five-month-old fetus is also acutely discriminating in its musical tastes, producing defined physical-emotional responses to different sounds. It can, for example, tell the difference between formal music and ordinary atmospheric noise. It is capable of learning the musical scale and of remembering lines from poems and songs that are frequently recited to it before birth.

According to similar studies, the measured and harmonious rhythms of Baroque composers such as Vivaldi, Bach, and Handel cause a prenate to enter a state of relaxation and contentment. The measured beats and simplicity of classical composers such as Mozart, Shubert, and Haydn produce a similar effect. When we come to the Romantic period, however, with its emphasis on deep emotion and strong tonal colors, the more intense works of composers such as Wagner and Bartok act as a kind of electrical shock to the prenate's nervous systems, causing it to kick and squirm about in the womb until the music stops. More agitating still is dissonant music—the compositions of, for instance, Stravinsky—and most disrupting of all to a prenate's musical ear, perhaps not surprisingly, are rock and roll, rap, and most commercial popular tunes. Indeed, music that prominently features percussion instruments such as drums causes the prenate to twist its body into positions that suggest it is experiencing discomfort and perhaps even pain.

One of my patients recently told me an interesting story: When his wife was pregnant, they would frequently sing two or three of the same Hebrew songs to their in-utero child. This songfest continued during the length of the pregnancy. Four years after their daughter was born, the mother was doing housework and singing one of the melodies she had chanted to her unborn child. Suddenly, the little girl joined in the song, repeating the lyrics verbatim along with the mother in her four-year-old way. Many years later, when the child reached adolescence, she found that she still remembered the words to at least two of these songs. The sounds that had been beamed to her while she was inside the womb were imprinted indelibly on her consciousness.

The sense of sight. An in-utero child's other senses, while not as developed as the auditory faculty, are also busily at work.

Though tightly shut, around the fourth month of gestation a child's eyes begin to become sensitive to the impact of light. The child literally senses light coming through the mother's body. If the mother is walking through a tunnel, the child perceives a certain kind of darkness. If she is standing in the full glare of the noonday sun, a sense of brightness is perceived. Too much light or too much darkness are both daunting for a prenate.

According to Verney and Kelly, even shining a powerful flashlight on a pregnant mother's stomach can cause a child to turn in the womb in an attempt to escape the overstimulating beams. Harsh blinking lights are worse, causing the prenate's heart to fluctuate in rhythm with the flashes. Though it has never been proved and is highly conjectural, some scientists even believe that mothers who spend a great deal of time at dance clubs during their pregnancy and who dance to powerful strobe lights, produce children with a tendency toward weak hearts.

Finally, by the time of delivery, a baby's optical skills include depth perception, a limited ability to focus, spatial separation, binocular vision, and discernment of color hues.[18] In short, while in the womb, a baby's eyes develop to the point where at birth it can focus and take in visual impressions, as evidenced by the fact that newborns fix their gaze quite intently—and intentionally—on the mother's face. As we shall see in the next chapter, this all-important locking of the eyes during the first minutes following delivery helps powerfully to stimulate the bonding between mother and child.

The senses of smell, touch, and taste. While there is little evidence to show that smell is learned in the womb—odors are, after all, airborne, and must be breathed in to be experienced—studies nonetheless indicate that prenates may become familiar with certain scents in the amniotic fluid surrounding them.

Research shows, for example, that newborns are attracted to the scent of their own mother's breast milk (not the breast milk of other mothers), even though these children have not yet been breastfed. Some researchers suggest that this ability originates from olfactory responses learned in the womb.

In a somewhat more sinister mode, studies likewise demonstrate that neonates who are exposed to small amounts of toxic PCB fumes—perhaps even to a single whiff—may experience a diminished sense of smell as adults.[19] At least ten recent clinical studies support this alarming statistic.[20]

As far as touch is concerned, a great deal more prenatal activity can be observed and measured. Many carrying mothers, for example, know that rubbing and caressing their belly in an affectionate way has a soothing influence on the child, according to Thomas Verney:

> By the seventh month of pregnancy the expectant mother will know the positions of her baby's head and feet. She can be encouraged to stroke firmly and repetitively from baby's head toward her toes, which is thought to accelerate the development of the baby's peripheral nervous system. More importantly, this message helps the pregnant woman and her partner make contact with the baby, enhancing the baby's feeling of being loved.[21]

Moreover, harsh, jarring sensations plus persistent tapping and overly rambunctious patting can alarm a child, conditioning it to be afraid of outside "attack." Mothers who are abused physically by partners or relatives during pregnancy have a two hundred times greater chance of miscarrying and a 300 percent greater chance of birthing depressed or mentally deficient newborns.

There is also evidence showing that an unborn child not only experiences physical pain, but also, starting from around the twenty-first week, actually cries in the womb as a reaction to this pain. Most examples, plus a majority of published studies on the subject since 1941, indicate that in-womb crying is triggered primarily by obstetrical procedure. "A hand entering the uterus to bring down a leg," writes David Chamberlain, "can conjure up prenatal tears. So can applications of forceps, injections of analgesia, inserting a catheter, or rupturing the amniotic sac."[22] In one birth drama, Chamberlain tells us, "a mother, two doctors, and three midwives heard a baby cry five different times over a twelve-hour period *before* labor began. They described it as 'a startling and awesome event.'"[23]

Audible crying before birth begins at around twenty-two weeks of gestation. The earliest recorded cries, Chamberlain points out, are from aborted fetuses from the twenty-first, twenty-second, and twenty-third weeks of gestation. Chamberlain writes that a baby is thus capable of crying for approximately half the time it lives in the mother's womb.[24]

Regarding the development of the sense of touch, using the delicate receptors of the skin, prenates start to make tactile contact with the fleshy, aquatic world surrounding them during the sixth week of gestation. Shortly thereafter, they stretch their limbs in earnest, reaching out with hands and feet to touch above and below their space.

By eight weeks of gestation, these movements are spontaneous and voluntary—not, as was once believed, automatic and reflexive. At this time sensations of touch appear in the hands, and at nine weeks of gestation, they appear in the soles of the feet. Around the same time, the fetus shows signs of skin sensitivity in the genital area. Ultrasonographers have even observed male children undergoing erections while sucking their thumbs at around fourteen weeks, evidence of early oral-genital sensory response and of a lusty plunge into self-pleasuring. By fifteen weeks of gestation, a prenate's entire torso is sensitive to touch.

What do all these developmental landmarks tell us in practical terms about an unborn child's learning potential? Primarily this evolving sense of touch allows a prenate to make overtures toward the outside world and to begin the process of interacting with its parents. We know, for example, that a prenate responds in a positive way to having its body stroked. When a pregnant mother rubs her belly in a loving manner, the child's pleasure response can be measured and graphed. On the other hand, unborn children exposed to invasive gynecological medical tests, such as amniocentesis, react with what can only be called a fight-or-flight response. Some prenates attempt to dodge the amniocentesis needles or wiggle away from their arrowlike tips. Others, presumably the more feisty and aggressive among them, box the needles away with hands and feet. Still others appear to watch, fascinated, as the needle probes around them.

These different responses to the same obstetric procedure tell us that an in-utero child's reply to invasive disturbance is powered not by knee-jerk instinct but by an individual psychological disposition expressing itself differently in different children: A prenate may express rage, terror, indifference, or curiosity. It is theorized that each of these reactions hints at traits of future personality. Further, these different responses are sparked not by the sense of touch alone, but also by a primitive sight reflex. "Though it cannot be explained easily," concludes one study, "prenates with their eyelids still fused seem to be using some aspect of 'vision' to detect the location of [amniocentesis] needles entering the womb, either shrinking away from them or turning to attack the needle barrel with a fist."[25]

These focused counter-punches are displayed by children before the parts of the brain responsible for emotional response are developed and long before the cerebral cortex, responsible for conscious thought, is operating at full throttle. This leads us to conclude that the brain and nervous system are busily reasoning and judging in utero before important parts of the brain are fully formed.[26]

As for the organs of taste, we know that by the fourth month of gestation the unborn child sucks if its lips are touched. If a bitter fluid such as iodine is introduced into the mother's amniotic fluid, the prenate grimaces and refuses to swallow the liquid. Evidence also shows that what a mother eats during pregnancy flavors her amniotic fluid and, consequently, her newborn's attitude toward eating.[27] For example, at around twelve weeks of gestation, the fetus begins to swallow some of the mother's amniotic fluid, committing its flavor to sensory memory. After the child is born, it recognizes the specific colostrum and the familiar taste of the mother's milk from previous contact with this fluid.[28] When presented the breast for the first time, the newborn thus suckles with a will and with a sense of familiarity. In the process, its survival potential is increased and the bond between mother and child is cemented.

An abrupt change of diet during pregnancy, therefore—say, from a heavy meat menu to a vegan menu—can confuse a prenate and upset future lactation patterns. For this reason, extreme dietary changes are discouraged in pregnant mothers who intend to breastfeed.

Finally, during early gestation, your child uses its developing senses to "practice" at real life—a learning process that humans follow for a lifetime. One example is fetal breathing. The motions that make up this process begin at ten to eleven weeks in the womb and mimic the lung movements newborns make when drawing their first breath.[29] A neonate also makes regular coordinated eye movements inside the dark womb, though there are no visible objects on which it can fix its sight. Such behaviors are thought to be trial runs, ensuring that in the first hours of life the real breathing that takes place and the real seeing will be familiar enough to newborns so that these functions can swing into operation automatically.[30]

Mental Health

Nature versus nurture? By the time a child emerges from the womb, how it has been treated by the outside environment—especially the love, hate, or indifference shown it by parents—has already wired its brain with a disposition toward happiness or alienation, adjustment or neurosis, kindness or hostility. Studies show that intelligence is affected by in-utero perceptions and that, contrary to long-time scientific belief, biologists now estimate that approximately fifty percent of a child's intelligence capacity may be developed by the time he or she is born.

Thus, despite earlier psychiatric thinking on the subject, children do not enter the world as "blank slates unwritten upon," as the English philosopher John Locke phrased it, and as many psychologists later adopted as gospel. Children's minds, hearts, and sensory apparatus are all written upon copiously by the time they are born—though in a language and with writing implements that we are just beginning to understand.

An in-utero child, for example, is constantly in rapport with its mother's hidden emotional life and with her deepest wishes and fears. It appears to know when the mother, and to some extent the father as well, are joyous, anxious, serene, or angry over the fact that it is being born in the first place. There is even a theory, backed by a small but growing number of studies, that spontaneous miscarriages in healthy mothers occur far more frequently in women who do not want their babies than in women who do. In such cases, it is hypothesized that the embryo, though barely formed, possesses ultrasensitive emotional antennae capable of tuning into the deepest moods and inclinations of the parents. If this embryo senses it is despised, it responds by slowing its biological functions until they cease, in this way engineering its own self-destruction. It chooses death rather than being unwanted—such is the importance of love to the prenate.

Chemical messengers. Many traits of childhood personality, including behaviors both naughty and nice, can be traced back to a pregnant mother's emotional frame of mind.

These traits begin as positive or negative chemical messages delivered through the placenta. They then take hold in the prenate, increasing in intensity and influence throughout gestation and birth and into childhood, adolescence, and adulthood. Because few parents make attempts to communicate with their unborn child and because in-utero learning is ignored by educators and mental health professionals alike, the cause of these positive or destructive behaviors usually goes undiagnosed. As a result, all of us become the recipients of our in-utero past.

"Because we don't consciously recall our prenatal and perinatal experiences," writes Swiss psychotherapist, Franz Renggli:

> we are inclined to repeat them continuously throughout our lives, to stage them again and again in our professions, partnerships, and with our children and friends. Emerson calls this *tendency recapitulation*. The more traumatic the beginning of our lives, the more we tend to recapitulate our vulnerability. Peter Nathanielsz [director of the Laboratory for Pregnancy and Newborn Research at Cornell University] showed that the conditions in which we develop in the womb profoundly influence our susceptibility to coronary artery disease, stroke, diabetes, and obesity in later life, reiterating the notion that people seek out therapy to resolve issues that originate with prenatal and perinatal trauma.[31]

A mother's attitude toward both her child and the world during pregnancy therefore conditions the mental as well as physical set of the emerging prenate. The entire process begins and ends with body chemistry. If, for example, during her child's gestation a mother regularly undergoes negative bouts of body and mind—anxiety, fear, shock, disease, extreme sadness—these states produce high levels of adrenal steroid hormones in her bloodstream.

Adrenalin is the fight-or-flight hormone manufactured by the adrenal glands when a crisis threatens personal safety. Secreted into the blood at the proper moment and in appropriate quantities, adrenal steroid hormones are just the tonic needed to help us stand and do battle or, when the odds overpower us, to vacate the premises energetically. But these hormones also rough up our physical equilibrium, causing changes in metabolism and body chemistry. Even in small amounts, they increase heart rate and blood pressure, make breathing patterns uneven and shallow, cause sweaty palms, and trigger a queasy stomach. If these conditions continue over a lengthy period of time, residual adrenal hormones accumulate in the mother's body and remain there like a stagnant pool, acting as a mental and physical toxin. Further, because mother and gestating child are linked in a complex chemical-physical web, high levels of adrenalin not only agitate the mother, but also pass through the placenta to generate copycat states of anxiety and stress in the child.

Because in modern life so many pregnant women consistently experience stress (from jobs, caring for other children, marital strife, money problems, psychological disorders), in-utero babies often find themselves under siege from these powerful adrenal stimulants and are duly affected. The crossfire can strike both from the mother's negative mental states and from her harmful physical habits such as smoking, drinking, workaholism, and drugs. Environmental contaminants also play a negative role.

Thirty years ago, Dr. Jeffrey A. Lieberman, as reported in *Fetal Growth and Development,*[32] observed an amazing correspondence between a mother's smoking habits and a child's learned anxiety. According to Dr. Lieberman's studies, whenever a pregnant mother thinks of lighting up a cigarette—simply thinks about it—the heart beat in her prenate increases dramatically and its anxiety levels shoot through the roof. It turns out that a fetus of six or seven months of age is aware enough and wise enough to remember that when smoke enters the mother's bloodstream, it becomes uncomfortable and perhaps agonized by the reduction of oxygen that tobacco causes in the blood. The fetus reacts with fear, just as if it was physically attacked.

Even more extraordinary is the fact that a prenate appears to be capable of reading the impressions running through its mother's mind: It knows when and if she is about to indulge her tobacco habit and it responds accordingly. Though it sounds like psychic mumbo jumbo, from a scientific point of view, the thought of smoking a cigarette most likely triggers certain chemicals in the mother's bloodstream that are then scanned immediately and understood by the prenate. Such rapport demonstrates the fundamental mind-body unity that exists between a mother and an unborn child.

The price of too much prenatal anxiety. What are the long-term effects of fear, anger, and stress on the developing prenate?

Over time, if an unborn child is exposed constantly to tensions through the mother, it develops a kind of permanent, free-floating anxiety, which, as we have seen, does not necessarily wane when the mother calms down. (We can recall, for instance, a prenate's reaction to audio overstimulation: The harmful effects linger after the sound itself passes.) If experienced too often, this anxiety increases, becoming a habitual response that, finally, is triggered independently of the mother's state of mind.

From this condition of escalating fretfulness and worry, a child finally comes to develop permanent feelings of distrust plus an unreasonable concern for its own safety. This concern translates behaviorally into acts of fear and violence expressed by the growing child (and later by the adult) as a means of self-protection driven by the philosophy of "better get them before they get me!"

Infant health is likewise burdened by maternal anxiety. If, for example, too many stress hormones are pumped into a fetus for too long, its chances of developing serious kidney problems during adulthood increase dramatically. In this particular script, high levels of cortisol slow down the in-utero growth of small tubules inside the kidneys (known as nephrons) that play a key role in the blood-purifying process. A child afflicted in this way grows up with a set of underdeveloped kidneys, which, during adulthood, can cause complications in blood filtration and in maintaining healthy blood pressure.

So much for prolonged anxiety—but how damaging to an unborn child are short-term episodes of stress? According to a number of studies,[33] the key to protecting a prenate from the ravages of stress depends largely on a mother's capacity to regulate her own arousal responses, especially anger and anxiety. Maternal efforts to alter these responses, we now know, exert a calming and organizing effect on mother and child alike.

The amount of damage done to a child by stress, anxiety, and depression, therefore, depends to a large extent on how diligently a mother works to neutralize these feelings and to overcome them. If a mother can return to a positive emotional outlook quickly after outbursts of anger or alarm, her unborn child can do the same.

Illness in the mother, though a definite anxiety trigger, likewise tends to leave no scars as long as the ailment is not serious or prolonged. It is difficult to say for sure, but it appears that the unborn child senses when negative episodes are transient or accidental and "forgives" the insults. This is especially true if the mother continues to harbor positive, optimistic thoughts toward her prenate while she is sick.

Finally, studies show that prenates who are continually under stress not only tend to develop into neurotic infants, but also later, as growing children and adults, experience a reduction in mental faculties: Their intelligence levels and learning capabilities can suffer dramatic downturns. In-utero children exposed to violence, especially abuse aimed at the mother, have a considerably higher incidence of psychotic ailments, childhood schizophrenia, and autism, than children who pass a relatively quiet gestation.

Nature versus nurture revisited. It is therefore evident clinically that as goes the pregnant mother so goes the child.

But why is this? Aren't all of us genetically designed and mapped out at conception? What do a parent's personal attitudes have to do with the formation of an unborn child's talents and abilities? Aren't physical makeup and personality development mainly predetermined by our genes?

Not exactly, says Dr. Bruce Lipton, one of the cutting-edge biologists currently at work on the question of nature (genetics) versus nurture (environment). In fact, Dr. Lipton insists, contrary to popular scientific notions of genetic determinism, though genes do control patterns that form a developing embryo, they have no innate ability to set the rules or to spin into motion the wheels of human development. Instead, genes must be activated and directed by signals received from the child's external world.

Therefore, the old medical model that our genetic inheritance cannot be changed, and that we are little more than heredity's pawns, misses the mark. On the contrary, Dr. Lipton maintains, the quality of impressions received in utero sets and resets the genes that comprise the human germ cell. This resetting ratchets up and down intelligence, emotions, and future talent levels on the scale of possibility, continually writing and rewriting the scenario of whom we will be when we are born.

Until the work of Dr. Lipton and his colleagues appeared, what's more, the notion that a prenate's perceptions influence its own genetic structure was unknown to biological catechism. Now, backed by a vast body of laboratory research, Lipton and his colleagues have challenged this dogma. Plus they have added an extra dimension: During pregnancy and even before, Lipton insists, parents act as genetic engineers for their own developing child. This act of creation depends largely on the parents' behavior and awareness, as well as on the raw perceptions of the unborn child. Lipton writes:

> The alternative perspective [to genetic determinism] expands upon the role of parents in human development. Those endorsing nurture as life's "control" mechanism contend that parents have a fundamental impact on the developmental expression of their offspring. In the nurture-controlled system, gene activity would be dynamically linked to an ever-changing environment. Some environments enhance the potential of the child, while other environments may induce dysfunction and disease. In contrast to the fixed-fate mechanism envisioned by naturists, nurture mechanisms offer an opportunity to shape an individual's biological expression by regulating or "controlling" their environment.[34]

What does all this mean in practical terms? First, as we have seen throughout this chapter and has been suggested throughout this book, a mother's affection and care—or the lack thereof—for her child sets the personality agenda for even an unborn infant. Lipton tells us:

> What the fetus is experiencing is the mother's environment. The fetus responds to her emotions and feelings exactly as she does. Why? It uses the nutrients it sucks from the mother's blood. The blood has more than nutrients in it. The blood has all the coordinating, integrating, communicating molecules that make the mother's body function. So the fetus is getting the same signals across the placenta. . . . The fetus can't see what's going on in the world. So what does it do? It relies on what the mother experiences. The fetus will adjust its physiology to what she sees. If she lives in fear, is that going to be growth-promoting to the fetus or not? No. It's going to change the genetics and the physiology of that fetus, so when it's born it's ready to live in fear.[35]

Reviewer Barbara Findeisen of *The Journal of The Association of Pre- and Perinatal Psychology and Health* writes:

> Previously, perception of the environment, particularly the mother's perception, was never considered to be a factor in genetic expression. However, as Dr. Lipton explains, it is the mother's perception of the environment during prenatal development that creates the environment in which the fetus must learn to adapt. The mother provides the information, and biology responds to it; when the environment is toxic or fearful, cells move away, there is a contraction and less growth, and the organism moves into defense and focuses on survival. But when the mother's environment is loving and joyful, the organism is engaged in growth and thrives. It is empowering for parents to know they can provide a healthful environment for their child even before birth.[36]

Second, and more groundbreaking in its implications, Dr. Lipton's findings, based on years of clinical research, also show that a mother and father's behavior alters the formation of their germ cells even before the sexual act and fertilization occurs—an alteration that takes place within the male sperm and the female ovum as many as thirty to sixty days prior to conception. This process is directly mediated by the parent's personal conduct: by what they think and feel during the period immediately before conception; by how they behave toward one another; by the way they act toward their friends, their enemies, their dog, their cat; by the foods they eat and drink; by what they read and watch on TV (or don't read and don't watch); by how they entertain themselves; by where they travel; by whom they socialize with; by how hard they work—in short, by every aspect of their lives.

"The parents, the persons who develop the sperm and the egg, are influencing the selection of genes in the germ cells even before they're released for fertilization," Lipton declares.

> The imprints are laid down before fertilization. It's the attitudes of the parents in the few months before conception that are selecting an imprint that will determine some very fundamental shapes and characters of their future baby. . . . How you are relating to the child or to the germ cell is actually changing the perception of the child. You have power over that developmental process. Because nurture is learned. . . . Long before you are ready to have a baby you should thus be thinking about this baby, and what you are planning with it. Your perceptions are influencing your own germ cells.[37]

Lipton's insistence that a parent's mind-set affects the child-to-be means that couples planning a family are well advised to consider living gently and wisely in the weeks before they attempt procreation. For this reason, it has become standard for most natural-birth counselors to champion the practice of optimism and positive thinking during this preparatory time. They encourage mutual kindness between mates; bathing each other in an atmosphere of contentment and love; warm socializing with trusted friends; good-humored play; getting plenty of rest; exercising regularly; laughing a lot; reading inspiring literature, poetry, and scripture; avoiding situations that conjure up fear and turmoil (such as hateful arguments or scary movies); playing with children and pets; eating nutritious foods; avoiding tobacco and drug use; drinking in moderation (or stopping entirely); avoiding prescription medications that are not necessary; and practicing wholesome spiritual disciplines such as yoga, tai chi, body work, psychotherapy, positive visualizations of the child-to-be, meditation, and prayer.

Studies show that all these behaviors alter positively the quality of sperm and egg, as well as strengthen the nervous and immune system of a child-to-be—which help produce a healthier, happier baby.

The physiological origins of violence. Finally, Dr. Lipton leaves us with an urgent warning that every community of parents, family, and friends is wise to heed. Inside the germ cell, he explains, there are twenty-three pairs of chromosomes, each with thousands of genes attached to it. These genes come in two varieties: one set derived from the mother and one set from the father. Only one of these gene sets can be used by the prenate. When one is blanked out, the other is allowed to express itself and vice versa.

Now these two varieties of genes, qualitatively speaking, are by no means alike. About two months before the female egg ovulates, it is activated and begins its final stages of maturation. During this last stage, an imprint is laid down concerning which genes are going to be selected. On what is this imprint based? Lipton answers: "The perceptions of the parents. The reason is this. There are two sets of genes: the ones in the father can imprint those in the sperm; in the mother they can imprint another larger set on the egg. The imprinting asks: Which of these two shall we negate or knock out? Which one should I activate?"[38]

These questions are essential as far as the temperament and even the destiny of the prenate are concerned—because maternal genes build a smaller fetus and one that favors, as Lipton phrases it, "love over brawn." Paternal genes, on the other hand, produce an organism with a larger musculature that is designed to fight and dominate its environment. Masculine genes also build a physical brain that is smaller and less well-developed than the brain generated by female genes; one that is more capable of surviving—physically as well as mentally—in a threatening environment, but is less capable of generating higher impulses of compassion, imagination, and care.

That's the trade-off in the genetic playing field: heart versus brawn. As Lipton points out, if we look at a fetus generated by male genes and one generated by female genes, we see that the forebrain, the part of the cerebrum necessary for higher thought and reason, is smaller in the male-gene prenate and larger in the female. Meanwhile, the hind brain (or mammalian brain) that is necessary for basic metabolic processes and fundamental survival reflexes is larger in the male than in the female. Again, this exemplifies brawn, protection, and brute force over nurture, serenity, and love.

How is the choice made between these two modes of genetic development? "In a supportive, nurturing environment this [the female-gene dominated fetus] is more of the embryo you would develop. If the parents live in a threatening environment that doesn't support their family or the future generation they will create an embryo that looks like [the male muscular, embryo with a smaller forebrain]."[39]

In other words, when a child is enmeshed in a "feminine" environment of parental love and peaceful surroundings, it opts for the female-based set of genes. In an atmosphere of anger, violence, and deprivation, Lipton insists, "parents create a child that can fight, yes. But this is going to compromise the intelligence of this child."[40]

He thus concludes:

How we parent our children today changes the future of evolution on this planet, and therefore our own children as the future parents. It is incumbent on us to know we have an active, dynamic role in making a better world. But we have to get out of our own belief system to do it. And to recognize we are not genetically determined but we actually influence every step of the way before conception, through development, and on into childhood. How we influence our kids can make superstars out of them with consciousness. Without consciousness we are probably doomed.[41]

TEACHING YOUR CHILD IN UTERO

Having established here that a prenate does indeed learn in utero, here are some parting thoughts on how you as parents can take full advantage of your unborn child's abilities.

The Role of the Father
The father can and should play an important part in the life of the unborn child. When considering pregnancy, we tend to think of the mother-child relationship alone. The fact is that fathers can also take steps to bond with their in-utero child and to help make the birth and subsequent child-raising tasks a happier occasion for everyone.

The relationship between the mother and father of an unborn child exerts a profound influence on the in-utero development of that child. Indeed, in some societies the connection between a father and his unborn child is so intense that he exhibits the same signs of pregnancy that mothers pass through—a phenomenon known in the Basque area of Spain as *couvade*. Fathers-to-be in these societies undergo morning sickness, feel a sensation in their bellies that can be described only as kicking, and, during labor, experience cramps and a pushing sensation. Such behavior can, of course, be construed as pathological, but only by the standards of our own culture. For other cultures, paternal behavior of this kind represents normal masculine empathy and is expected. Such reactions prove the degree of closeness that is possible during pregnancy between a father and his soon-to-be-born child.

In our own society, one way in which fathers can participate eas-ily in the rite of pregnancy is simply to be as kind, loving, and supportive of the mother as possible. Though this help comes to the child in an oblique fashion, the father's tenderness and good intentions are communicated. They also raise the mother's spirits and with them her immune system response, protecting her health and her daily state of mind and, in the process, supporting the growing child. The image that best exemplifies paternal care is that of a circle: mother feeds child while father feeds mother while mother feeds child. The ring is unbroken and continuous.

A father is advised to make as much contact with the unborn child as possible by stroking the mother's stomach, talking to the child, singing aloud, and meditating upon the child's future welfare. One father I know tells his unborn infant a little story every day: a five-minute narrative about how nice the world is and what a splendid time it will have in this place. Studies show that a placid and affectionate father's voice exerts almost as calming an effect on the child as that of the mother.

While in bed at night, a father can hold the mother closely, generating a physical warmth and mutual affection that passes directly to the child. This sensation of affectionate parental touching appears to be like honey for a prenate, helping it attain deep states of comfort, security, and relaxation. In a recent study of thirteen hundred children, it was estimated that those women who experienced intense antipathy or neglect from their husbands were 237 percent more likely to bear a psychologically damaged child than women who experienced a happy, nurturing partnership.

Be Wary of Ultrasound

Though perhaps a bit off the subject of parent-child intrauterine bonding and connection, but nevertheless de rigueur for many pregnant women in the West and resulting in problems for some prenates, a caveat should be issued at this point on the medical procedure of ultrasound.

Ultrasound was developed originally during World War II as a shipboard method for detecting enemy submarines. Since that time, it has been used by the medical profession with gratifying success to diagnose serious diseases such as cancer. It remains a valuable and much needed medical device.

During the 1950s, it was also discovered that ultrasound scans of a pregnant mother in the fifth month of pregnancy could predict possible infirmities in a child. In some cases it can detect uterine bleeding, scope out twin or breech births, and perform several other useful pediatric functions. Today, prenatal ultrasound is used routinely on millions of mothers-to-be.

But pregnant women should be careful. Statistically speaking, prenatal ultrasound is not a highly accurate device. In Australia studies show that ultrasound failed to detect early problems in 40 percent of women, and some estimates place diagnostic success as low as 10 percent or less. In more cases that are not much talked about in the medical profession, doctors have received a false positive diagnosis and aborted the fetus, only to discover afterward that the prenate was healthy.

More worrisome is the fact that ultrasound waves warm highlighted areas of the fetus and, in the process, potentially cause tissue damage. A second unpleasant effect, *cavitation,* results in small pockets of gas vibrating and in some cases collapsing and causing subsequent tissue collapse. This then produces a range of chemicals, some of which are highly toxic to the developing fetus. One study of cavitation shows that cell abnormalities produced by exposure to ultrasound lodge in human tissue and can then be passed down from mother to child for several generations. Rat studies likewise show that ultrasound occasionally damages the myelin sheath covering the nerves of the spine. In the human organism, when the myelin sheath is harmed, multiple sclerosis may result, along with several other neurological problems.

The upshot is that in many cases prenatal ultrasound is only partially effective as a diagnostic tool and at the same time carries statistically small but nonetheless real dangers for mother and child. Though many physicians order ultrasound as a matter of course today, parents-to-be are advised to think twice before using this method routinely unless there is already a known cause for concern.

Explore In-Utero Learning

Finally, there is much to be gained from working with other parents who are exploring and practicing in-utero learning. Since 1980, organized programs have been developed to help parents communicate with their unborn child and to teach them exercises, both physical and meditative, that expedite in-utero learning.

Your exploration can start by asking friends and natural health care professionals about prenatal learning courses in your area, by reading local children's magazines and handouts in midwives' offices and health food stores. *Mothering Magazine* (a good source in general) sometimes advertises organizations that specialize in this field. Better yet, search the Internet for information on the subject and for the names of prenate learning groups near your home.

The largest program in prenatal stimulation in the world today is located in Caracas, Venezuela, where, under the direction of psychologist Beatriz Manrique, six hundred families have been involved for more than ten years in prenatal learning experiments, which include testing babies for cognitive and perceptual skills after birth. Reports David Chamberlain in his paper "Early and Very Early Parenting":

> Test results revealed the advantages of prenatal stimulation in virtually every category over the entire time period, including verification of superior auditory and speech development, motor skills, memory, and intelligence. Because of such positive results, the government of Venezuela has decided to make the program available throughout the country.[42]

These studies, Chamberlain concludes,

> . . . have proven what few believed in 1980: (1) that babies in the womb are alert, aware, and attentive to activities involving voice, touch, and music (2) that babies benefit from these activities by forming stronger relationships with their parents, and their parents

with them, making for better attachments and better birthing experiences, and (3) that these babies tend to show precocious development in speech, fine and gross motor performance, better emotional self-regulation, and better processing. . . . These are the gifts of early parenting.[43]

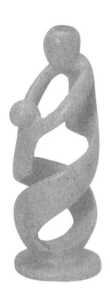

4
Birth
Labor and Delivery

Imagine what might happen if the majority of women emerged from their labor beds with a renewed sense of the strength and power of their bodies, and of their capacity for ecstasy through giving birth. When enough women realize that birth is a time of great opportunity to get in touch with their true power, and when they are willing to assume responsibility for this, we will reclaim the power of birth and help move technology where it belongs—in the service of birthing women, not as their master.

CHRISTIANE NORTHRUP, M.D.,
WOMEN'S BODIES, WOMEN'S WISDOM

"IT'S AN INTERESTING AND, I think, instructive idea," a midwife once told me, "to think of a child's entire in-utero life cycle from conception to delivery as part of a single prolonged birthing process. A baby starts to be born the moment it is conceived. It is never too early to get ready for the event."

As we have seen, a great deal of scientific evidence backs up this notion: conception, pregnancy, and birth are part of a single creative continuum.

At the same time, giving birth is an entirely separate event from pregnancy, a real-life passion play that is different from all that has come before and that is rich in its own ecstatic drama and biological pageantry. Never in all their lives are newborns' sensitivities keener and more receptive than at the moment they pass from darkness to light, gazing on the faces of their fellow human beings for the first time and receiving thousands upon thousands of sensory impressions from the great garden of the world that suddenly surrounds them.

In general, the sudden current of perceptions that floods a child's consciousness at the moment of birth comes in two basic flavors: positive and negative. In the modern birthing room there is little gray area in between. Nine times out of ten, a newborn's experience is agitated or ecstatic, violent or serene, heartless or heartfelt—depending on the setting, the person who delivers the child, the parents' behavior, and the medical methods used in the delivery. The impressions taken in at this critical moment, what's more, are literally branded into a newborn's subconscious, hereafter affecting everything they think, feel, and do: their decisions, moods, work, play, intelligence level, learning capacity, social skills, love of life, the way they will parent their own children—everything.

According to a growing number of medical professionals, many of whom we will hear from in the pages that follow, birth is a prime determiner of who we are and how we behave. Its affects last forever.

A WOMAN'S EXCLUSIVE DOMAIN

Over the millennia, the control and overseeing of childbirth has always belonged to women. Traditionally, female relatives and female friends attend the birth, and a female midwife delivers the child. Delivery takes place in a woman's bedroom or in a familiar domestic setting. In many instances a *doula*—a female helper—is part of the delivery team, performing nonclinical birthing chores, providing emotional support, and helping to talk mothers through the ebb and flow of labor. Based on eons of human experience, everyone agrees: in matters of childbirth, women know best.

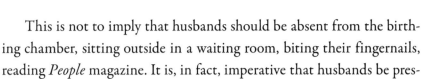

This is not to imply that husbands should be absent from the birthing chamber, sitting outside in a waiting room, biting their fingernails, reading *People* magazine. It is, in fact, imperative that husbands be present at the event, providing loving support and encouragement throughout the delivery. In most traditional cultures—those in which certain practices and beliefs are passed on from generation to generation—a central position is provided for the father in the birthing place.

Despite the importance of a father's role, however, it is the mother who invariably takes center stage during birth. It is from her body that the newborn child emerges; it is the mother who must go through the agonies and ecstasies of parturition. The first earthly form a newborn sees is the mother's face. It is the mother who places her child to the breast and who gives this new little being succor for the first time. All the while, the child remains tied to the mother's body via the umbilical cord, a palpable symbol of the mystical maternal attachment that will last a lifetime. From this perspective as well, the birthing chamber is and always has been the sanctuary of the female.

For millions of years, the female psyche has been hard-wired with an understanding of what to do at birth and how to do it. Most women (though not all) appear to be born with an innate sense of how to cooperate with nature during pregnancy and birth and how to provide robust, loving nurture once their child is born. By means of maternal instinct and by tangible faculties such as heightened senses, hormonal stimulation, chemical cues, intuitive body wisdom—and most of all, from thousands of years of genetic imprinting—a mother possesses all the tools necessary to birth her child. In her, the package is complete.

"Birth is a woman's work," insists Dr. Marshall Klaus of the American Society of Pediatricians. "When she has no female relatives or friends who feel comfortable supporting her, she needs a doula. When birth is truly normal this way everyone benefits—mothers, babies, fathers, and society."

Since the beginning of time, this concept, that women are the gatekeepers and guardians of the childbearing realm, has been part of a society's wisdom . . . in all societies, that is, except our own.

THE BEGINNINGS OF THE MODERN
MEDICAL MODEL OF CHILDBIRTH

During the late seventeenth century and to some extent before, fantastic discoveries in biology, chemistry, and mathematics shook the world and helped to create a new view of life and of the universe around us.

It seemed that as the centuries passed, science was learning the true anatomy of the physical world—first, from a Newtonian world machine perspective, then on an atomic and subatomic level. In the process, people began to believe that science could and would solve all the problems that beset the human race. Just as a higher power had once been considered the sole keeper of the worldly order, now science appeared to step in and take over as determiner of human fortune, becoming eventually a veritable substitute for God, with the scientist acting as surrogate priest.

This brave new world of hope and technology soon took hold with special vigor in the field of biology and in biology's proudest offspring: the healing sciences. By the late nineteenth and early twentieth centuries, using scientific methods of testing and inquiry, medical researchers began to gain remarkable insights into how the human body really works. In late nineteenth-century France, for example, Louis Pasteur formulated the germ theory of infection, changing forever the face of the medical world and saving billions of lives. He also invented the process of pasteurization.

In 1895, Wilhelm Roentgen discovered the X-ray. In 1922, insulin was synthesized, prolonging the lives of countless diabetics. Anesthesia, modern nursing practices, hygiene, sanitation, surgery, and nutrition all advanced with seven-league boots following the Civil War, and by the early twentieth century, cures for diphtheria, syphilis, typhoid, yellow fever, and dozens of other acute bacterial diseases freed humanity from demons that had preyed upon it for eons. Finally, in 1928, due to the tireless labors of Sir Alexander Fleming, the greatest curative marvel of all time was invented, the medical magician's pièce de résistance: antibiotics.

It is difficult to explain with full justice the amazement and worshipful gratitude people felt toward science during the late nineteenth and early twentieth centuries. Medicine, they now assumed, would ultimately discover a cure for all forms of human illness. Eventually, the world would become free of disease. Medical science was coming to know all of nature's secrets.

By the middle of the nineteenth century, the modern hospital also made its appearance. True, in the beginning the notion of hospitalization instilled enormous fear in many people. Going to a hospital was a terrifying experience for many, and the common thought of most people, especially the elderly, was, "If I go to the hospital, I'll never come back." Nonetheless, science marched on, and by the early twentieth century the belief that slowly but surely took hold was that every discomfort was a disease that should be cured via the medicalized hospital.

This notion—that every bodily discomfort is a medical problem that requires a physician's attention—was soon translated into the belief that childbirth itself, along with pregnancy, is a health crisis and a physical illness; that pregnancy is, in fact, a dangerous medical condition; and that the only foolproof way to help pregnant mothers "get well" is for them to give birth in a sanitized, sterilized hospital environment using drugs, medical equipment, anesthesia, and a qualified medical specialist to perform "the operation." Birth and delivery, once the exclusive domain of the female, were thus taken from women entirely and given over to the male-dominated medical profession. By the end of World War II, the overseeing of pregnancy and delivery had become an exclusively male institution.

In the process, especially during the 1940s and 1950s, medicine began to introduce strange new birthing theories based on medical models rather than on the experience of women themselves. It should be said that no other civilization, even the most backward and decadent, had ever dreamed of such theories and ideas—which soon became strict, obstetric gospel in the physician's office and birthing room. Indeed, doctors in Europe and America alike, confident they were ushering in an enlightened era in obstetrics, now informed the world that new scientific findings had proved the inarguable validity of the following dictums:

✤ Pregnancy is a hazardous medical condition. As a result, childbirth should take place in a hospital environment, where female patients can be kept under constant medical surveillance and supervision. Birth at home, even under the supervision and care of a trained obstetrician, puts both mother and child in dire risk of losing their lives.

✤ Childbirth is by definition an excruciatingly painful event. The agonizing and inescapable convulsions experienced during delivery are an inevitable "symptom" of the pregnancy-birthing "disease."

✤ The notion that women possess an inborn, instinctive knowledge of childbearing is a myth. The male doctor always knows the best course of action to take during pregnancy and delivery, despite what the mother's body and intuition may be telling her. At the same time, the readouts from medical devices ultimately override even the opinions of the doctor, determining all the final decisions made in the hospital room.

✤ To prevent complications and to help deaden the unbearable pain, mothers-to-be should be fully or partially anesthetized. During the 1940s and 1950s, it was common practice to drug a mother into oblivion at the time of delivery, then to keep her unconscious until several hours after the birth.

✤ For reasons of safety, c-sections are required in a large number of deliveries. The need for episiotomies is even more common and mandatory.

✤ Lying flat on the back in a hospital bed (thus defying the laws of gravity that have always expedited the newborn's delivery) is the only position that ensures that the mother births successfully. Sometimes a mother must even be strapped down or otherwise restrained. Today, unusual delivery positions, such as squatting or bearing on all fours, are practiced mostly by uneducated peasants in backward third-world countries.

❖ A mother should never move from the supine position during labor and birth. She must remain entirely still. Walking around during labor, stretching, standing up, talking to other people, sitting in a chair, eating—all such activities are potentially harmful to mother and infant alike.

❖ During the moment of birth and in the days that follow, a newborn remains in a kind of unconscious cocoon, utterly insensitive to its surroundings. Bright lights; loud noises; extremes of temperature; brisk handling; having its nose and mouth suctioned out immediately after birth, then being weighed on a cold metal scale; long periods of separation from the mother; a slap on the rump to stimulate breathing; the hubbub of attending strangers in the birthing room; and the burning pricks of inoculation all exert little or no influence on the newborn's somnambulant consciousness.

❖ After delivery, newborns should immediately be separated from their mothers for "hygienic" reasons. At birth, children are highly susceptible to the legions of germs that swarm around them and must be kept in isolation in a quasi-sterile nursery for their own sanitary protection. Newborns should then be kept in isolation from their mothers for much of the time during their hospital stay. The mother, despite her deepest needs and yearning to hold her newborn child, should be allowed access to her offspring only during designated hours as specified on the hospital's nursery schedule.

❖ Breastfeeding can malnourish children and even damage their health. Synthetically manufactured commercial formula is far richer and more nourishing than mother's milk and is the only food fit for hungry newborns.

❖ The father has no place in the birthing room and should be isolated from the delivery process entirely. After delivery, his handling of the baby must be managed even more closely than that of the mother.

✤ Midwifery is a dangerous and outmoded practice. It has caused innumerable unnecessary deaths and in the best possible world should be outlawed entirely. (Indeed, even today midwifery is banned in several states.)

In short, over the years the medical profession, assuming a position of absolute knowledge and unchallengeable authority, has slowly but surely disempowered parents from having any say whatsoever in the birth of their own child. With these firm beliefs, father and mother alike, obviously incapable of comprehending the vast risks and complexities of medical delivery, became reduced to the status of spectators, to passive participants in a highly hazardous and terror-inspiring surgical procedure known as giving birth.

Thus the irony: In the name of providing safety and comfort for mothers-to-be, the most unnatural and frightening birth scenarios ever devised on the face of the earth were now considered the norm.

A NEW ERA DAWNS

During the early post–World War II years, these dogmas and dictums of the medical community began to be reevaluated by a number of medical professionals. Change was clearly in the air. The first signs of parental reempowerment arrived with the coming of a concept known as *natural childbirth.*

This change began to a large extent with Dick Read, a British obstetrician who for many years delivered babies in the London slums. After a long practice, Read came to certain conclusions that ran counter to all contemporary obstetric wisdom. The anguish and panic of childbirth, he claimed, are not an organic part of the birth process. Terror of delivery and birth pangs are grossly exaggerated by the medical profession and are fostered and even encouraged by the profession itself and are passed from woman to woman, magnified in the process with each telling.

The antidote to this manufactured crisis, Read claimed, is to return to more organic and traditional methods of birthing and delivery. True, there are times during a difficult birth when anesthesia is required or when emergency measures must be taken. In such circumstances, all conventional medical interventions should be brought to bear immediately. He proposed that given a sound baby in a sound mother's womb, however (which is the case in 95 percent of births), there is absolutely no reason why childbirth must be such an intimidating process. On the contrary, giving birth should be the most joyous experience ever undergone by a man and woman during the course of their lives. Nature has even designed it this way, said Read. All the biological and psychological tools are at hand, inherent in the female psyche and physical makeup. These tools must simply be recognized and put to use. Nothing new or extraneous is required.

Here though, is the rub. In order to take advantage of the many maternal aids and intuitions nature has bestowed on women, mothers-to-be must cooperate with rather than resist the forces of nature. As we know, mothers and fathers of the twenty-first century have been taught so thoroughly to believe that the medical model of birthing is not only the best model, but also the only model that most parents accept the common obstetric indignities without a peep. Never mind that these indignities, in a majority of cases, not only are unnecessary, but also create the very problems they are designed to relieve.

But, many may still ask, what about the matter of pain? How can a mother rely on nature's wisdom alone while contractions are washing over her like molten waves, causing her to writhe in suffering, tension, trauma, delirium, and dread? Again, replied Read, the current-day medical management model is to a large extent responsible for creating this writhing. While presiding over countless births throughout the years, he observed that when natural methods are used in delivery, a vast majority of mothers experience relatively low levels of pain and fear, and in many cases there is no pain at all. Contrarily, in the modern-day hospital room, the system seems designed from the ground up to make birthing patients feel cornered, helpless, abandoned, and entirely at the mercy of outside forces.

We can imagine for ourselves this very moment, the amount of angst generated today during a typical hospital birthing experience: cold hospital-room walls, stainless steel medical equipment surrounding the bed, the shaving of private parts, the injections of drugs and antibiotics, the inducing of labor with hormones, the premature breaking of the water, the tests, the IV, the prohibition of eating and drinking, the blood drawing, the anesthesia, the constant electronic-field monitoring and beeping of machinery, forceps delivery, masked doctors and nurses moving about the mother's bed like phantoms. Added to these factors is the mortifying body-shame felt by a mother when she is peered at during this most vulnerable of all moments by doctors, nurses, and young medical students; and the threats mothers have been warned of so thoroughly from the moment of conception: birth complications, hemorrhaging, induced labor, breech birth, c-sections. Plus, there is the pervasive atmosphere of worried and hurried professionalism displayed by the stern-visaged physicians and specialists.

How could such an accumulation of daunting input not cause mothers to become overwhelmed with anxiety? How could such influences not create an internal chemical and hormonal chaos within a mother that leads to unbearable physical tension and to unmitigated emotional terror? In short, Read insisted, all the dire warnings concerning what one doctor termed "the bloody nightmare of bringing a baby into the world" are part of an unnecessary and harmful system invented over a hundred years ago by a male-dominated obstetrics profession to maintain control over the birth process and the birthing parents. The real problem is not the "disease" at all; it is the "cure." We can recall the old vaudeville line: "The operation was a complete medical success, but the patient died."

Writes Read in his seminal book, *Childbirth without Fear,*

I . . . picture a crowd of men in white coats and large horn-rimmed glasses seeking fame and fortune searching for a weapon with which to protect all women from an enemy, which in 95 percent of cases does not exist, and their chosen method of protection is to risk the life of the woman and her baby by using that weapon upon them, and upon the enemy, which they erroneously presume to be present.[1]

WHAT IS NATURAL CHILDBIRTH?

What exactly are the techniques that Read pioneered and that have been developed with such finesse and expertise since his time? Further, how do these techniques work, and how do they differ from (and why are they better than) the conventional medical model? Most significantly, why is natural childbirth so important to a child's early development and to the mental and physical health that children will someday experience as adults?

While several encyclopedia-sized works could (and have been) written to address these questions, once explained, even in the most general and concise way, the basic concepts of natural childbirth tend to strike an immediate chord in a majority of parents-to-be. Many ask why they were never before told about these options. These methods seem very attractive to parents-to-be: once the details are explained, they become excited over the prospect of natural childbirth.

First, these concepts are readily understandable and easy to put into practice—far easier, it should be said, than the practices used in the conventional medical model. Second, practitioners of natural childbirth are privy to a vast array of new scientific knowledge that supports its approach to labor and delivery and that disproves a number of the supposedly inviolate principles on which the modern medical model of birthing is based. Also, the principles of natural childbirth hearken back to a wisdom that is ancient and forgotten: a knowledge buried in the feminine collective memory that is crying out to be heard once again. Finally, while this ancient inner voice calls continually to women on an intuitive level, new scientific data developed in labs and studies around the world helps us better understand the miraculous preprogrammed hormonal orchestration that takes place within a woman's body during birth just as clearly as we understand other fundamental body processes such as digestion and respiration. This new data, much of which is unknown to the public at large and to parents-to-be, shows us how and why nature itself—as opposed to the medical intervention model—is the best of all birthing guides and teachers.

Before we discuss natural childbirth itself, let us look at aspects of this new science and, in the process, ask the following questions:

1. What are the fundamental biological processes of birth and how do they work?
2. What has science discovered in the past several decades concerning the physiology of birthing?
3. How does this new information support and buttress the concepts of the new parenting?

The Hormonal Orchestra at Work

The following information, based largely on the writings of Sarah J. Buckley,[2] explains how a mother's preprogrammed chemical birthing blueprints are read spontaneously and deciphered during pregnancy, labor, and birth. It also demonstrates the fragility of these blueprints, explaining why interference with a mother's natural biological engineering can sabotage the entire course of a birth, damaging both mother and child in the process.

One of the most critical aspects of this maternal biology, as explained by Buckley and others in the field, begins with hormones.

The four hormone groups. In a nutshell, hormones are protein telegrams that carry chemical messages and instructions in the blood, telling certain organs of the body what to do and when to do it.

During childbirth the primary hormones responsible for activating and controlling all other hormone systems are the basic sex hormones: progesterone and estrogen.

While pregnant, the amount of progesterone produced in the placenta increases ten to eighteen times. Estrogen levels rise more than a thousand times.[3] These two primary chemical activators, progesterone and estrogen, are in turn responsible for mobilizing the so-called four major birth hormone groups, which control the detailed chemical interactions that take place during labor and birth. When permitted to function on their own without external interference, these hormone groups perform a majority of the work necessary for a successful delivery:

- Oxytocin: a pituitary-mediated hormone that causes uterine contractions in women, increases sexual desire, and produces the ejection of breast milk, sometimes known as the "hormone of love"
- Beta-endorphin: a hormone that induces pleasure, a sense of well-being, natural analgesic qualities, and feelings of emotional transcendence during birth
- Adrenalin group: a hormone excreted from the adrenal glands that increases metabolism and other stimulating chemicals in the blood of both mother and child
- Prolactin: a hormone that stimulates breast milk and lactation in new mothers

During birth, estrogen increases the number of uterine oxytocin receptors,[4] while estrogen and progesterone together activate the beta-endorphin hormone that acts as a natural opiate painkiller, preparing the pathway in the brain and spinal cord for a more comfortable labor.

Most interesting, when all these chemical substances work in concert, one of the least understood aspects of natural birthing takes place: ecstasy. This natural "high" is not due simply to the psychological joy of giving birth. It stems from the hormones themselves that flood the bloodstream of mother and newborn, generating profound changes in the brain and neurological systems of both. These ecstatic sensations give a mother a sense of her own personal power and physical strength, plus an intuitive understanding of her newborn's needs. Such realizations, in turn, foster a joyous mutual dependency between mother and child, ensuring that the mother provides care (including bonding and lactation) and thus protects the baby's survival.

These four hormone groups—inducing love, transcendence, stimulation, and mothering—are all produced in the limbic system, that part of the brain from which our emotions come. During labor they build to a critical mass, peak at birth, then reintegrate into the mother and child's systems in the post-birth hours and days that follow. Once birth and the time after are completed, these substances, having served their purpose, return to normal levels within the blood. All parts work like integrated and perfectly balanced instruments playing together in a symphony orchestra. Mammalian animals of every kind have followed this blueprint without any type of assistance since the beginning of time. Spontaneous labor in a normal woman is an event marked by a number of processes so complicated and attuned so perfectly to each other that any interference will only detract from their optimal character. The only thing required from the bystanders is that they show respect for this awe-inspiring process by complying with the first rule of medicine: *nil nocere*, "do not harm."

Disrupting the balance. What happens, though, if this hormonal dance, so complete on its own and so independent of any need for human help, is interrupted? When such disturbances take place, the hormones turn against the mother, in a manner of speaking, producing a dysfunction in the labor process.

If such dysfunction is triggered by a medical intervention, which is usually the case, this often makes another medical procedure necessary to right the wrong caused by the first intervention. Sometimes another procedure must then be performed to keep the spiral of chemical imbalance in check, eventually creating layer upon layer of dysfunction in a chemical system that is engineered by nature to handle the labor and delivery process entirely without outside help.

As Read so cogently pointed out, this already confused process is thrown into further imbalance by distractions in the hospital environment itself: bright lights, loud noises, surrounding machinery, the mother's mental anguish that has been churned up by fears implanted in her mind. All these jarring factors add to the further disarray that takes place within the mother's hormonal equilibrium. The irony of all this uncalled-for tinkering, moreover, is that after medical methods have thrown off the working of a mother's internal chemistry and the application of further interventions to repair the problems caused by these methods, mothers end up enduring an unnecessarily prolonged, fraught, and painful delivery, then, absurdly—and commonly—coming away from the process feeling gratitude toward the medical establishment for being "saved."

A Closer Look at the Four Hormones

To better understand the details of how the four birth hormones cooperate during birth, let us take a closer look at the workings of each hormone group during moments of labor and delivery.

Oxytocin. This "love hormone" is secreted into the bloodstream during the acts of sexual activity, orgasm, birth, and breastfeeding. It is also manufactured in each of our systems when we are engaged in pleasant social situations and at moments of gladness and appreciation, making it a hormone of altruism as well as of sexual activity and birth.[5]

During birth, a baby releases large amounts of oxytocin. This substance is transported through the placenta into the bloodstream, where it circulates freely back and forth between mother and child. Research shows that this exchange excites a mother's uterine muscles, giving added "oomph" to the final, powerful birth contractions (sometimes referred to as the *fetal ejection reflex*) that help push a child out of the womb with maximum force and efficiency.[6]

If, however, this oxytocin release is disturbed during delivery by certain obstetric interventions, it can produce a slowing of contractions. Misreading the situation, doctors may then consider this slowing to be an indication that the mother is too weak to push the baby out on her own. More interventions are deployed to "help" the mother deliver—at times including what would have otherwise been an entirely unnecessary c-section.

Other effects of oxytocin: When the baby's head begins to crown during birth, the "stretch receptors" in a woman's vagina are stimulated, initiating the release of oxytocin in large quantities. After birth, as the baby touches and licks the mother's breast, this oxytocin buildup helps the mother's uterus contract, protecting her from postpartum hemorrhage. Other oxytocin triggers that produce similarly benign effects include skin-to-skin and eye-to-eye contact between mother and baby.

In the mother, oxytocin levels peak during and after delivery, then drop gradually over the next sixty minutes. The newborn's oxytocin supplies reach maximum levels thirty minutes after birth, then subside during the next hour, causing both mother and baby, as Buckley describes it, to be "[b]athed in an ecstatic cocktail of hormones, including oxytocin, the hormone of love"[7] in the first hour following birth.

Finally, during pregnancy, oxytocin enhances the utilization of nutrients within the body and helps mothers conserve energy. Scientists now understand that oxytocin also lowers anxiety response during pregnancy and lactation, fostering feelings of well-being in pregnant and breastfeeding mothers and making them more resistant to alarm and nervous tension. During breastfeeding, oxytocin likewise aids the smooth ejection of breast milk (the so-called letdown reflex) that is released in pulses as the baby suckles. During the months and years that follow birth, oxytocin levels help mothers feel more relaxed and at one with their child during the on-going process of breastfeeding.

Beta-endorphin. Beta-endorphin has been called the natural internal opiate. Secreted in all of us whenever we feel pain and psychological pressure, beta-endorphin reaches exceedingly high blood levels during pregnancy, birth, and lactation.

Similar to addictive opiates such as heroin and cocaine, beta-endorphin induces feelings of pleasure, euphoria, release, and dependency. During labor, its levels reach those produced in male endurance athletes who run at maximum speed on a treadmill.[8]

These high levels of endorphins help mothers transmute pain into pleasure and enter the altered states of consciousness and ecstasy that are nature's gifts to birthing women. Babies in the process of birth also receive endorphins from the surrounding placental tissue, and from here these substances flow back through the umbilical cord into the mother. This process has led researchers to speculate that early cord cutting may "deprive mothers and infants of opioid molecules designed to induce interdependency of mothers and infants."[9] More on this later in this chapter.

Adrenalin group. Adrenalin, along with associated corticosteroid hormones, is one of the major hormones produced in response to stress and prepares the body for "fight or flight." It is also one of the primary forces during childbirth, occurring in sudden bursts to stimulate the fetal ejection reflex. Along with many other functions, these bursts help to "wake up" the child in the womb, supply needed energy for both mother and child, provide mental focus for mother and child, and help the child assume proper delivery position in the birth canal.

During birth, report doctors Irestedt, Lagercrantz, and Belfrage,

> The mother experiences a sudden rush of energy; she will be upright and alert, with a dry mouth and shallow breathing and perhaps the urge to grasp something. She may express fear, anger, or excitement and the adrenal rush will produce, in concert with oxytocin, several very strong contractions, which will birth the baby quickly and easily. The baby experiences a rush of the adrenal group, particularly noradrenalin at the moment of birth, occasioned by pressure on

the baby's head. In addition this group of hormones helps prepare the lungs through helping to absorb the amniotic fluid from the lungs.[10]

Problems start, however, when a mother becomes overstressed. As we have seen, this condition takes place during medical interventions and when mothers are exposed to intimidating hospital conditions. For example, high adrenalin levels in the first stage of labor inhibit oxytocin, thereby slowing and in some cases even stopping the process of labor. All mammalian creatures, including human beings, have a hard-wired ability to oversecrete adrenalin. This is designed to provide the mother with the ability to slow labor in the face of danger, thereby buying her time to find a safer birthing location.

High levels of adrenalin also reduce the blood flow to the placenta, and thus to the child. They contribute to prolonged labor and in some cases to abnormal fetal heart rate. Too much adrenalin in a stressed mother's system can likewise create postpartum problems, including lethargy and depression. Over the long run, children who are born with unnaturally high adrenalin levels tend to be cranky, colicky, and less mentally focused than children born in calm environments.

Prolactin. This hormone prepares a mother's breasts for lactation, playing a major role in milk synthesis, milk production, and breastfeeding. Also known as the "mothering hormone," one researcher describes prolactin: ". . . A key player in the organization and behavioral adaptations of the maternal brain, prolactin levels rise during pregnancy, helping to organize the mother's brain towards motherhood. After birth, prolactin levels are directly controlled by the suckling intensity, duration, and frequency."[11]

Here are some of the known psychological and physical effects of prolactin on the brain:

⚶ It enhances a mother's devotion to the needs of her baby.

- $ It produces a type of anxiety that activates maternal vigilance and encourages a mother to place her baby's needs above her own.
- $ It prompts benevolent maternal behavior toward the child.
- $ It suppresses postpartum fertility, hence preventing a mother from becoming pregnant too soon after birth.
- $ It reduces body temperature.
- $ It increases secretions of oxytocin.
- $ It increases endorphins and other natural opiates manufactured by the body.
- $ It helps adjust the sleep-wake cycle, increasing REM sleep, or deep sleep, for nursing.
- $ It induces a state of natural analgesia and pain relief.
- $ It plays a role in maturing lung function in the unborn fetus.

Needless to say, when prolactin is inhibited by medical interventions, both a mother's milk production and a child's sucking reflex are diminished. When breastfeeding is disrupted in this way, most if not all of its benefits are lost to both mother and child.

ALL ABOUT NATURAL CHILDBIRTH

The overview here of birthing physiology and of the new scientific knowledge we now possess sets the stage to understand and appreciate the modalities practiced in natural childbirth. But what, specifically, are these modalities and how do they differ from conventional delivery techniques? How do they work and why do they work?

- $ To begin, natural childbirth encourages home birth, and if home birth is not possible, it considers as a second best birth in an independent birthing center or in a hospital birthing center.
- $ Natural childbirth also prefers that delivery be performed by

a qualified midwife or by a (preferably) female obstetrician who practices natural birthing techniques.

❧ Natural childbirth likewise suggests that drugs, sedatives, epidurals, anesthesia, hormones, medical monitoring machines, and other accoutrements of hospital birthing play a minimal role in the delivery, if they are used at all.

❧ The process also discourages c-sections and episiotomies, substituting more gentle methods to coax a child through the process of birth.

❧ It stresses relaxation, freedom from fear, open dialogue among all involved members of the birthing party, birth education for parents, help from other women, and the loving companionship of husband and wife during delivery.

❧ It asks that labor and delivery take place in a quiet, friendly environment that is chosen and arranged by the parents-to-be. It encourages water births, labor in a Jacuzzi, immediate mother-child bonding, and alternate birthing positions.

❧ It insists that a newborn remain with the mother immediately after birth rather than being carted away to a baby ward. It insists that the newborn be allowed to suckle at the mother's breast the moment it emerges from the womb.

❧ Natural childbirth likewise introduces the father back into the process of nativity. It makes him a primary player in the drama of his own child's birth, allowing him to help the mother push through her pain and endure her contractions and to provide loving emotional support for his spouse during and after delivery.

Introducing the Midwife

As a health care professional once said to me, "Prostitution is supposed to be the world's oldest profession, but there is one that's even older: midwifery."

In times long past, the midwife was celebrated as the bringer of life to the tribe, the clan, and the village. Within the community she was looked on as an exalted person and sometimes as a sacred one. Even today her name in French—*sage-femme*—and in German—*weise frau*—means "wise woman."

With the coming of modern medicine's takeover of pregnancy and birthing practices, the profession of midwifery fell on hard times. In 1900, 50 percent of all births in the United States were presided over by a midwife. Thirty-five years later the number had dropped to 12 percent. By 1940 it was less than 5 percent. Midwives continued to practice their arts quietly in poor urban areas of the country and in rural farm districts. Yet by the middle of the twentieth century, it appeared that midwifery was being swept away by the iron hand of the medical establishment, along with a host of other long-proven natural healing modalities.

Even so, despite everything the government, the American Medical Asssociation, the medical profession, the drug companies, and the various corporations that profit so richly from medicalized obstetrics did to abolish midwifery, this ancient profession has made a return to the birthing chamber, transformed now into a science as well as an art. (For specific information on finding and choosing a midwife, see the resource section.)

Choosing the Best Method and Location for Natural Delivery

Natural childbirth is not a single monolithic system but instead is made of a spectrum of options that range from homebirth with a midwife to hospital birth with a doctor accompanied by a few childbirth amenities.

Hospital natural birthing center. First on the list of hospital options is the natural birthing center located within a conventional hospital setting. This apartment-like facility is separate from the standard hospital maternity ward and is often located on a different floor. It is set up to accommodate midwife-assisted birth along with the personal requirements and requests of the parents-to-be.

The rooms in such a center are large and decorated comfortably—they are a cross between a living room and a bedroom. Furnishings include large, queen-sized beds in which mothers can assume different positions constantly and move about at will. A typical birthing center has pictures on the wall; rugs on the floor; dining tables; easy chairs; a small refrigerator; an attached, private bathroom; often, a Jacuzzi in the birthing room; and many other homelike amenities—all of which, needless to say, are more likely to foster an undisturbed birth, allowing nature's blueprint of cascading hormones to flow as planned. Such a birthing center is opposed to the cold walls and looming medical machinery of standard hospital delivery rooms. Also provided is a range of facilities for attending family and friends, and mothers are allowed to keep their babies with them for the duration of their hospital stay.

As for birthing equipment, all medical apparatus is kept hidden until it is needed. In our own birthing experience at Roosevelt Hospital in New York City, a large, rather attractive painting covered part of the wall behind the bed. If the picture was slid to the side on a track, revealed was the medical machinery stored behind it. In our birth the apparatus was not needed except to make some minor sutures after our son was cradled safely in our arms.

You can call your local hospital to ask if they provide natural birthing facilities. If they do not, you may have to search, as we did, until you find qualified natural childbirthing personnel and a center that fits your needs. Hospital birthing rooms are an attractive alternative to home delivery not only because they offer the benefits of nurse-midwife delivery, natural-birthing methods, and people-friendly surroundings but also because immediate medical care is only a hospital floor or two away should a serious problem develop.

Independent birthing center. Another attractive natural birthing alternative is the freestanding, out-of-hospital birthing center. It provides a wide range of conventional medical facilities should they be needed, including a doctor on call and immediate ambulance service. At the same time, the emphasis is on midwifery; natural birthing; parental empowerment; a relaxed, homey atmosphere; and family-centered care.

A room in a freestanding birthing center can be downright luxurious. Over-stuffed couches, designer wallpaper, Jacuzzis, eat-in kitchens, bathrooms with dual showers, and other pleasures of hotel and home are common features. A center usually requires weekly birth-education classes for parents, and family members are welcomed to take part in the birth, provided this is part of the parents' birth plan. Finally, all the modalities of natural birth are practiced at independent birthing centers: The mother uses a midwife, she delivers in whatever way and position she chooses, she decides for or against drugs and episiotomies, she avails herself of natural relaxation procedures, she walks about freely during labor, she breastfeeds her newborn, and she keeps her baby with her from the moment of birth to checkout time.

Thirty-seven states currently license independent birthing centers. The expenses of having a child at these centers are considerably lower than at a hospital, and costs are now covered by a number of insurance companies.

Water birth. Most independent centers (and some hospital birthing centers as well) now offer water birth as an alternative to birthing in bed.

It consists of laboring and delivering in a deep tub or pool filled with water and heated to a temperature of 97° to 100°F. The mother usually enters the tub when her contractions reach two to three minutes apart and her cervical dilation reaches around four to five centimeters. Once the mother is immersed, the water-induced buoyancy helps her to relax; to move about freely; and, if she so wishes, to deliver her child unsupported by another person. Meanwhile, the warm water eases and speeds up contractions, stimulates blood circulation, and reduces pain.

When the time comes for delivery, the newborn slips out of the birth canal and enters the water directly. Because it has been floating in a watery environment for nine months, the warm currents are familiar and serve as an ideal transition medium from womb to world. Further, because a newborn is still connected to its mother via the umbilical cord, it receives all the oxygen it requires while underwater.

Once it is out of the womb, a newborn is then allowed to float freely underwater for thirty seconds to a minute; then it is removed from the tank; its nose and mouth are wiped clean; and, for the first time, it is exposed to the sounds, sights, and touch of the world around it. This sensory stimulation sends a "time to breathe" signal to the child's brain, and most water-birthed babies start to inhale and exhale on their own, as do all naturally birthed babies. At this point, the mother brings the child to her breast, the baby begins to suckle, and the process of bonding begins.

How safe is water birth? Studies have been done in the United Kingdom to determine the risk factors involved. Results show that water birth is as safe and even slightly safer than a conventional lying-in birth. One study carried out between 1994 and 1996 in England and reported in the *British Medical Journal* shows that among 4,029 babies born in water, the mortality rate is 1.2 percent compared to a control group in which the mortality rate is 1.4 percent giving water birth a small edge in safety.[12] We should note incidentally that labor in a Jacuzzi is not the same as water birth. Many mothers prefer to spend part of their labor immersed in the soothing waters of a Jacuzzi, with their spouses in attendance supportively, and then to deliver their child in bed. In general, warm water is highly recommended for a laboring mother to relax and divert her and expedite her contractions.

Conventional hospital delivery with selected natural methods. Finally, because of a growing demand, parents who wish to deliver in a more or less conventional way are nonetheless offered certain natural childbirth methods by an increasing number of hospitals.

One such option, for instance, is Labor, Delivery, and Postpartum Care (LDP). In LDP, labor and delivery take place in a private room with a labor and delivery nurse backing up the doctor. Ahead of time, parents work out a birth plan with their doctor that suits their needs and inclinations. This plan often includes aspects of natural birthing, depending on the hospital's facilities and tolerance to natural birthing techniques. A caution: This plan can also be a wolf in sheep's clothing— that is, high-tech birth dressed up in humanistic trappings.

Birthing classes. Classes in birth education are also offered at most hospitals today. These methods include the Lamaze or Bradley systems, which provide techniques for breathing and relaxation during labor. Parents-to-be learn about the stages of birth, the mechanics of labor, how dilation takes place, and intervention options for both pain and assistance. Much of the information taught in birth education classes pertains to natural procedures and to methods that allow a husband and wife to work together as a bonded birthing team.

Home Birth. A majority of home births today are performed by a mid-wife in the warmth and security of the mother's own bedroom. Though there are obstetricians and general practitioners who perform home birth, they tend to be few and far between.

How safe is home birth? This will come as a shock, but statistically, there are six times more infant mortalities in hospitals than in home births. This unpleasant little secret, as well as the surprisingly large number of iatrogenic (doctor-induced) deaths that take place in hospitals, is kept from parents-to-be by just about everyone in the medical profession.

Despite the outcries of some members of the medical profession, then, when it is practiced properly, home birth is as safe or safer than hospital delivery. An important factor: while advances in hygiene, sanitation, medical knowledge, delivery techniques, scientific understanding, and levels of education go a long way toward ensuring that a home birth is successful, it is the midwife herself who ensures that the birth is both a positive and safe experience. Certified midwives, for example, are highly trained at handling home-birth emergency situations of all kinds. Indeed, due to the intensive training she receives in this area, a competent midwife knows as much and sometimes more about birthing safety than the average obstetrician—and if a problem does arise that requires intensive medical care, midwives are expert at setting up protocols for immediate evacuation to a nearby medical facility.

According to C. Hafner-Eaton and L. K. Pearce at Oregon State University, ". . . literature shows that low-to-moderate risk home births attended by direct-entry midwives are at least as safe as hospital births attended by either physicians or midwives."[13] Writes H. C. Woodcock, et. al, in a volume on home delivery: "Planned home births in Washington appear to be associated with less overall maternal and neonatal morbidity and less intervention than hospital births."[14] Numerous other scientific studies can be cited concerning the safety of home birth.

A final note of caution: If at any point in the pregnancy cycle a serious complication does arise, it may be prudent to cancel your home birth plans and move the delivery to a hospital. If such a problem does present itself, consult with your midwife and health care professional concerning the most judicious course of action.

CREATING A BIRTH ENVIRONMENT THAT WORKS FOR YOU

One of the primary benefits of natural birthing is that parents are given the option to choose both the place of birth and the birth ambiance they most prefer.

Music is a must for many parents. Some prefer sounds pulsing with energy; others like their music gentle and contemplative. Parents-to-be may wish to sing, play an instrument, hear jokes, watch a video, even dance. One couple I know spent their hours of labor alternatively playing "Monopoly" with family members, then sitting in a circle with friends and relatives, holding hands, and singing songs to the in-utero baby. In a natural birth environment, all the body senses should be involved and rewarded during labor.

Some mothers tend to become passionately hungry during labor. Eating and drinking are encouraged at this time, so remember to stock the birthing room with favorite foods and drink. If a mother relaxes in a hot tub or participates in a water birth, she will also tend to dehydrate after an hour or two. Plenty of liquids are in order to counteract this. In fact, mothers-to-be should always stay well hydrated throughout labor no matter which birthing methods they chose.

Relaxation is the key to pain reduction in birth and to a joyous mental attitude.

Relaxation prevents a pregnant woman from releasing too much adrenalin into her bloodstream and hence into her child. (Adrenalin, you will recall, produces the fight-or-fight mechanism in a fetus, causing a surge of anxiety in the fetus and sometimes slowing or even shutting down the birth process itself.) Full mind and body relaxation is thus a critical goal in any natural childbirth scenario. During labor, for example, many mothers enjoy a full-body massage or a foot rub, and most midwives and doulas are proficient at these and other body arts.

Some mothers find that a low-light environment with candles burning, incense in the air, aromatherapy oils wafting, and fragrant ointments on the skin are all wonderfully conducive to a sense of safety and inner ease. During labor, still other mothers practice meditation, either alone or with their husbands and friends. Over the past decade, meditation has indeed come to the forefront as one of the most powerful methods we have for helping birthing mothers to focus and relax, and thereby to reduce anxiety, increase pain tolerance, enhance well-being, and even bolster the mood and energy level of the about-to-be-born child. It is no accident that the word *medicine* and the word *meditation* are derived from the same Latin root meaning "to cure."

According to recent clinical studies,[15] meditation boosts the production of several hormones critical to successful labor and delivery. Regular meditation sessions, for example, trigger an increase in the hormone DHEA, which in turn brightens mood and reduces nervous energy. Extra supplies of melatonin are also manufactured during meditation, heightening the relaxation response in the mother and the immune system response in the child. Levels of serotonin, a critical mood-enhancing and tissue-healing neurotransmitter, are likewise elevated during these sessions, along with supplies of endorphins, critical for pain relief and pleasure enhancement.

Contrarily, when labor is induced with drugs such as Pitocin, the reverse situation occurs. Writes Robert Newman, president of the organization Medigrace, which has studied the medical effects of meditation for more than a decade, "Pitocin, a common labor-inducing agent, and other medical interventions, are known to reduce or stop endorphin production and make inevitable the use of chemical pain blocks. Endorphin production is important to a woman in avoiding the risk of medical interventions and in developing psychophysical confidence in her natural abilities in childbirth."[16]

Extensive research on meditation carried out over the past years at the University of Massachusetts Medical Center notes incredibly that the frequency of cesarean section in meditating mothers is reduced by 56 percent, while the use of epidural anesthesia is lowered by 85 percent.[17] Still another benefit includes improvement in the quality of the mother's contractions. Writes Newman:

> All together, melatonin, serotonin, endorphins, and increased pain-management skills, all attributable to meditation, enable women to receive contraction sensations without risking pain-killing chemicals and anesthesia. Meditation also allows women to experience the joy that comes from using innate ability, actualizing realization potential natural to childbirth, the potential for human development, and illumination latent in the childbirth process.[18]

Finally, as a supplement to various forms of joyous labor play, many mothers enjoy the amorous caresses of their partner during these tender moments. Kissing, long embraces, fondling, nipple play, and bathing or showering together are highly recommended during labor, and all can be accommodated in a well-designed birthing room or home bedroom. What's more, during labor, sex itself is an age-old practice for stimulating the induction of contractions. "Prolonged and continuous nipple stimulation," writes Nancy Griffin in *Mothering Magazine*, "results in the natural release of oxytocin and is a proven nonmedical method for inducing labor. The release of semen into the cervix during intercourse can promote cervical ripening because semen contains prostaglandin, a hormone partially responsible for cervical softening."[19]

This range of life-enhancing exercises, all mightily taboo in a conventional hospital setting, also serve a deeper purpose than simple stimulation and diversion for mothers-to-be. When performed in the spirit of optimism and joy, these activities promote a profound sense of serenity and partnership with a mother's body and soul. This pleasurable mental state automatically generates sensations of security, joy, empowerment, love, and most of all, freedom from fear—all time-proven recipes for neutralizing the pain and terror that have become such a standard part of conventional hospital delivery.

In her book *Women's Bodies, Women's Wisdom,* Christiane Northrup, M.D., writes; "Many women describe birth in natural settings as erotic. Ina Mae Gaskin, in her classic, *Spiritual Midwifery,* writes that women need to be loved in labor, to be treated like Goddesses."[20] Northrup makes the sage point that the birth of a baby consummates the prior acts of intercourse, conception, and gestation that initiated and nurtured the final birthing process. With the birth of the baby, the circle of life is now brought around fully. Northrup tells that after delivery some mothers choose to present the baby formally to the father as a sign that the cycle of creation has come full circle and is now complete. In traditional Jewish practice, for example, the male child, before being ritually circumcised, is carried on a pillow by the mother and presented to the father with the words, "I have carried this child for nine months. Now take our son and circumcise him according to our laws." Other cultures worldwide follow similar rituals.

HAVING LOVED ONES
IN ATTENDANCE

Still another benefit of natural childbirth is that the husband becomes a necessary part of the birthing procedure, and, if the birthing couple so chooses, parents, grandparents, siblings, relatives, and even close friends can become part of the charmed circle.

If you do intend to have extra company while giving birth, be sure to discuss this matter with your partner, making sure both of you are in full agreement on all arrangements and on the fact that added onlookers can in some cases mean added stress.

Once you find agreement, advise your birthing professional of your plans well in advance of the birth date so that the delivery room can be set up to accommodate visitors. Another piece of advice: be sure that the friends or family you invite are fully and lovingly supportive of the style of birth you chose. This is no time to prove anything to anyone or to have a well-meaning relative blurt out advice or criticism suddenly. On this most happy of days, you—mother and father—are the central decision makers. Everyone else is an invited and privileged guest at your own ceremonial rite of passage. Be sure to keep it this way.

BIRTHING POSITIONS:
THE DECISION IS YOURS

The story is told that the great sun king, Louis XIV of France, took both a scientific interest and a prurient pleasure in watching ladies of his court give birth. Because it was easier to study these proceedings when a woman was lying flat on her back in stirrups than when she was squatting or standing up, Louis mandated that all women of the court henceforth give birth in the supine position. Thus was born a tradition in the West that has been with us ever since.

Whether or not the story is true, certainly the flat-on-the-back supine position has become standard operating procedure in the delivery room over the past seventy-five years, and this because . . . because of nothing. It is a fashion, it is "the way it is done"—and, coincidentally, this posture makes the delivery process easier for attending physicians.

The fact of the matter is that the supine position defies gravity, making it more difficult for a laboring woman to push during contractions and for a child to slide easefully down the birth canal. There is also much research to show that a forceps delivery is rarely necessary when women are allowed to assume nonsupine postures such as squatting. Indeed, over the centuries women have assumed whatever birthing position was most comfortable for their needs. This choice, in turn, depends, in part, on how the child is seated in the womb and the mother's anatomical structure. Common birthing positions include sitting, squatting, half-squatting, on all fours, lying on a side, and in some cases standing up. In a natural birth environment laboring mothers are also invited to walk about the room and change positions constantly: they can stand up, sit down, lie down, bend over, lean back, squat, sway, rock, undulate their hips when contractions come, lean against a helper, or allow themselves to be propped up by a partner or doula or other women—all the while talking and working in intimate contact with their partner and helpers.

What is the best birthing position to assume? Interestingly, scientific evidence supports the notion that during labor and delivery, the unborn child communicates constantly with its mother through a little-understood exchange of hormonal messenger molecules, providing the mother with various birthing instructions in a silent visceral language. It is theorized that one of the most significant suggestions a child transmits to the mother's consciousness at this time is the posture that will optimize its positioning in the birth canal and maximize ease and speed of delivery.

So what is the best birthing postion? It is best to follow body wisdom in this regard and to let instinct decide. There are no right or wrong birthing postures. Whatever position works best for a mother-to-be should be the position of choice in natural childbirth.

WHAT TO KNOW ABOUT DRUGS AND ANESTHESIA

The paradigm of painful childbirth—the notion that giving birth is an excruciating, high-risk peril rather than a joyous epiphany—has recently received a great challenge from the enormous body of scientific evidence that has become available increasingly over the past five years through professional journals that can be found on the Internet as well as from the press and exposure in the media.

It is common knowledge, for example, that when a delivering mother's muscles go into spasm and her mind is gripped with anxiety—as happens typically in the hospital delivery room (and as women are conditioned to expect through the passing on of the modern medical myth)—this tension not only produces pain, but also serves as a catalyst, magnifying all other pains, sometimes to an intense degree. A serene, undisturbed birth environment, therefore, along with the positive emotional expectations offered by the benefits of natural birth, encourages a mother's body and spirit to be fully centered. As a great deal of research shows, this comfort and lack of fear reduce a laboring woman's suffering level substantially, sometimes to a surprising and occasionally amazing degree.

Midwives are trained in a number of modalities that reduce pain levels in a natural way. Visualizations, meditation, herbal potions, hydration, and relaxation techniques are common tools at a natural delivery. So are baths, showers, immersion in a Jacuzzi, autohypnosis, hot- and cold-pack applications, massage, breathing techniques, pressure-point therapy, and targeted exercise regimens. New natural methods of pain relief, such as sterile water injection, can be employed. Gentle, supportive dialogue plus loving touch from a partner, midwife, or doula relieve a woman's pain substantially and help her cope without recourse to machines and drugs. Finally, should the pangs of delivery become too intense, midwives in a number of states are legally allowed to administer mild sedatives—rather than epidurals and powerful medications that disrupt contractions and increase anxiety.

Many mothers-to-be may ask, "Will there be pain during natural childbirth?" The answer is yes, probably some and perhaps a good deal—but perhaps there will be none at all. Every mother and every birth are different and there are no guarantees, but it is important to remember that pain is part of the natural process. It is the gateway through which all human beings must pass into the world, a kind of initiation ceremony, a challenge to be met by both mother and child.

The natural birth process that Dalit, our son Kesem, and I experienced was, as Dalit offers, much in this vein. She said after the delivery, "Actually, the contractions were much like a painful period cramp—but perhaps three to four times more intense. Each one lasted only thirty seconds or so, and then I rested until the next one."

Moreover, many women report that once they are experienced, even the sharpest contractions are, in a sense, there for a reason. Mothers perceive this pain not as an enemy but as an aid in the pushing and delivery process, and many say they would feel somehow cheated if they had to go through birth numbed from the waist down by chemicals, cut off from the rhythms of their own bodies. They are also mindful that once administered, pain-killing drugs go directly from the placenta into the fetus in less than a minute, triggering an increase in fear-inducing adrenal hormones and causing the child to be born in a state of utter panic. More alarming, a large number of women who take pain-killing drugs during labor report a decreased maternal attraction toward their newborn plus an increase in postpartum depression.

As for the safety of birthing medications, studies reveal that pain-killing and anesthetic drugs can and often do trigger medical problems in a newborn, at times inducing hypoxia (lack of oxygen to tissue), asphyxia (suffocation), and in certain cases damage to the child's brain and central nervous system. No drug in the canon of pain-killing chemicals has yet been invented that is known to be safe for a newborn child.[21]

The Epidural

This popular form of pain control, used in approximately 50 percent of hospital births today, calls for injecting an anesthetic into the epidural spaces in a mother's middle and lower back. This medication then numbs the nerves that control lower body function. The so-called spinal, an older form of anesthesia, calls for injection of chemicals directly into the spinal cord in the same manner as an epidural. Spinals are more short acting than epidurals unless they are administered as a combined spinal-epidural.

For some mothers, epidurals block the pain entirely. In almost all cases they provide a substantial level of relief—though in the process they also deaden the delivering mother from the waist down, making her oblivious to the miraculous creative act taking place in her own body.

An epidural can consist of several types of drugs, most of them cocaine derivatives such as bupivacaine/marcaine, ropivacaine, and lidocaine. These powerful anesthetics deaden the motor and the sensory nerves, ceasing all lower-limb movement. In the process, studies show, epidurals produce a harmful effect on the hormones of birth, inhibiting specifically the hormone-induced birth euphoria produced by beta-endorphin and oxytocin, which are so necessary for an ecstatic delivery.[22] (Indeed, modern medicine's reliance on epidurals may stem in part from its resistance to altered states of consciousness of any kind, which our cultural consensus denies and therefore looks upon with suspicion and dismissal.) The irony of this: our culture is becoming increasingly addicted to the use of mind- and state-altering substances such as alcohol and drugs.

When under the effects of an epidural, moreover, the high levels of oxytocin and the adrenal hormones that occur at the final stage of delivery are lowered significantly due to a numbing of the stretch receptors in the lower vagina that trigger natural oxytocin production. This numbing compromises the crucial fetal ejection reflex, lengthening the birth process, sometimes for hours, and often causing the birth to end with a forceps delivery.

Further complicating the situation are the effects of epidural drugs on the newborn as well as the mother. First flooding the mother's bloodstream, these drugs then pass straight into the child's brain, where they remain for longer periods of time than normal after the umbilical cord is cut, in the process compromising the child's respiratory and cardiac adaptations at the moment of birth.

In an interesting study from France, after giving epidurals to laboring sheep,[23] researchers observed that the animals failed to display normal mothering behavior toward their offspring after birth. Seven out of eight of these animal mothers showed no interest in their offspring for at least thirty minutes. Human studies likewise demonstrate that mothers given epidurals spend less time with their babies in the hospital and that the larger the dose of drugs they receive, the more aloof they are toward the child[24]—thus beginning, through a natural progression, the mother-child distancing we see so commonly in our culture and which becomes the "detached" style of parenting practiced by so many parents.

These shifts in relationship and maternal inattention may reflect hormonal dysfunction or drug toxicity. There is also evidence to suggest that babies born under the influence of epidural drugs have diminished suckling reflexes and breastfeeding capacity.[25] A recent study shows that healthy full-term babies born under the influence of a maternal epidural resist breastfeeding even before the time of the hospital discharge.[26] This phenomenon causes many new mothers to say, "I tried, but I just couldn't breastfeed." These mothers then give up on breastfeeding entirely, missing out on nature's special gift to mother and child. See the next chapter for more on breastfeeding.

Besides throwing the birth hormones out of kilter, epidural anesthesia involves major medical risks. Nausea, itching, heightened blood pressure, changes in fetal heart rate patterns, neonatal sepsis (blood poisoning), an increase in the need for cesarean birth, and induction of fever are all possible complications. For the mother, epidurals can also cause long-term urinary incontinence, as well as paralysis and spinal nerve damage. An article in the *American Journal of Obstetrics and Gynecology* tells us:

> Research reveals that although an epidural can completely block labor pain for most women, it is also associated with significant risks that many women may not be aware of. To make informed decisions about its use, women should be aware that epidural analgesia is likely to alter the normal processes of labor and birth, resulting in the routine use of other interventions to monitor, prevent, or treat associated side effects.[27]

Because a majority of parents do not read medical journals as a matter of course, however, most of them, like most of the general public, have never even heard about this alarming possibility.

Finally, many mothers who birth naturally express gratitude that their children have entered life drug-free, fully aware of the amazing sights and sounds surrounding them and of the loving parents standing nearby and welcoming them to the world with awe and open arms. Delivering mothers often tell us that if it was not for the total clarity and sense of personal empowerment engendered through transformative pain, both they and their child would have missed out on this ecstatic moment of awareness that comes only when mother and child are awake fully at the critical moment of birth.

STANDARD HOSPITAL BIRTH
PROCEDURES AND INTERVENTIONS

Though the space-age technology that surrounds mothers in a hospital delivery room is no doubt dedicated to fostering safer births, many conventional birth procedures and interventions are now coming under serious scrutiny. Within this criticism, there is a truth: These procedures can and do save many lives during emergency situations, and herein lies their inestimable value. Yet in an overwhelming majority of normal birth situations, hospital interventions are not only unnecessary, but also often cause physical and psychological complications. Following, we look at some of these standard procedures and examine the possible complications.

Fetal Monitors

An electrical fetal monitor (EFM) is designed to measure both a child's heartbeat and a mother's level of hydration. Here is how it works: First, a fetal scalp electrode is attached to the baby's head. At the same time, a catheter is threaded into the mother's uterus to measure intrauterine pressures. In the process, the mother is forced to assume a rigid, on-the-back position and is then obliged to remain immobile in this posture for long periods of time, pinioned to her bed in a web of straps, tubes, and belts. As the hours pass, this confining posture causes painful back spasms, muscle cramps, nausea, and claustrophobia, not to mention the anxiety generated by being hooked up to and, in a sense, tied up by a beeping, flashing, robot.

Are fetal monitors necessary? In an article published by the *New England Journal of Medicine,*[28] studies show that the use of fetal monitoring, when compared to listening to the heart rate directly, does not improve birth outcome. The article goes on to say that the routine use of EFM, compared to the traditional method of listening to the baby's heartbeat with a fetoscope, actually causes more problems than it prevents. Similar studies come to similar conclusions: The Friends of Homebirth organization states that "Each of these interventions in a normal labor has its own set of risks. . . . And none of these procedures has ever been proven to be more advantageous in eliminating complications or to produce healthier babies."[29] In eight randomized clinical trials, the article tells us, prenatal mortality was not reduced to any extent by the use of fetal monitoring. At the same time, in some cases fetal monitoring is known to generate a need for cesarean sections.[30]

Breaking the Water

In today's hospital delivery room, obstetricians frequently—and prematurely—break the water sack surrounding a child in utero.

Usually, there is no compelling reason to perform this procedure. It is done simply to speed up the delivery process and to get on with it. At the same time, because the possibility of uterine infection increases dramatically once a child's protective water bag is broken, this intervention automatically sets a time limit on the delivery schedule and produces an artificially rushed and hectic birthing atmosphere.

Inducing Labor

Another frequent hospital birth scenario takes place when labor is induced in pregnant women by means of chemical agents. This process is performed routinely by injecting synthetic oxytocin (the drug Pitocin) into the birthing mother's bloodstream, thus causing the mother's uterine contractions to occur more frequently and in closer sequence than under normal birth conditions.

This process is not without its hazards. It is known by scientists, for example, that speeding up contractions gives a newborn less time than normal to recover from the loss of blood and oxygen that occurs when its placenta is so rapidly compressed. Buckley points out, "Oxytocin augmentation stimulates uterine contractions, but has minimal effects on cervical dilation; compared to a natural labor this creates the possibility of 'failed induction,' where the cervix fails to dilate and a cesarean becomes necessary."[31] It is also known that women who receive synthetic intravenous oxytocin are at higher risk of postpartum hemorrhage than mothers who give birth naturally.[32] Synthetic oxytocin (Pitocin) can likewise trigger an increase in the resting tone of the uterus. This increase produces abnormal fetal heart rate patterns and fetal distress, which, statistically, increase the need for cesarean section.[33] In some instances, an increase in resting tone can also lead to uterine rupture.

Still another negative aspect of synthetic oxytocin: when Pitocin is introduced into the mother's bloodstream in the form of a steady intravenous flow rather than via rhythmic pulses (as occurs naturally with oxytocin), this break in biological continuity sends a signal to the child as well as to the mother to shut down the internal production of natural oxytocin. It is held by many researchers that when a newborn produces natural oxytocin at the time of birth, it is literally training itself to secrete its own love hormone. In the child's future, this hormone will be secreted as part of the natural course of things, providing the grown child with a capacity for intimacy, self-regard, and closeness with other people.[34] When the production of natural oxytocin is interfered with, however, as during an induced labor, there is a good deal less of the natural love hormone available to both mother and child at the time of birth. This diminished supply extracts a heavy toll, producing a less attached mother and a more aloof child. A newborn's future capacity to produce natural oxytocin is likewise affected and diminished, sometimes for life. For this reason, some researchers claim that the epidemic of low self-esteem and the inability to become intimate with others, which brings so many to the therapist's office today, in some cases can be traced back to the inhibition of natural oxytocin that occurs when childbirth is artificially induced.[35]

The Episiotomy

Another technique overused widely in the hospital delivery room, an episiotomy calls for the surgical cutting of the perineum muscle located between the mother's vagina and rectum. The purpose of this procedure is to enlarge the vaginal opening, ensuring that a child can pass through an unobscured opening when the vagina appears to be incapable of stretching to a wide enough circumference.

Statistically, episiotomies are medically necessary in less than 20 percent of childbirths. In many hospital settings they are nonetheless a routine part of delivery: many babies do, in fact, appear to have difficulty squeezing through the pelvic passageway, and most obstetricians are taught in medical school that the vagina is an inelastic organ that possesses very little "stretch ability"—that is, it cannot expand adequately on its own during labor and, more often than not, requires a bit of surgical assistance.

In fact, however, the human vagina is both highly elastic and highly flexible. The fact here: the process of dilation simply progresses at its own speed in its own time, not adhering to anyone's "stretch schedule" but its own. As a result, in the hurried operating-room environment many physicians perform episiotomies not because they are medically necessary, but because these obstetricians simply don't know any better or because time is short. (There are, after all, other deliveries scheduled for the same day, and delivery-room space is always at a premium in a hospital.) In the process, many doctors ignore the fact—or are ignorant of it—that in a vast majority of births the vagina eventually widens on its own to adequate size, providing safe passage for the child and necessitating zero surgical procedures for the mother. It is simply a matter of letting nature move at its own pace and of allowing time.

It is interesting that births presided over by midwives require far fewer episiotomies than those performed in hospitals. Midwives are trained to deliver babies without recourse to incisions or cutting, thus they know a number of "tricks" to promote dilation in natural ways. They are also taught to be patient—to bide their time and to let nature follow its own course so that a mother is allowed adequate time to push her baby out on her own in a slow, rhythmic, unhurried way. Midwives know that in a vast majority of cases, when the baby seems stuck in the birth canal, the mother's vagina is simply enlarging at its own pace and will eventually expand fully to accommodate the child's size. With careful waiting and watching, the newborn will come out on its own, free and clear.

Midwives also know that a small amount of tearing during the delivery process is sometimes inevitable, but these small vaginal tears are trivial and easy to repair, whereas the wounds sustained by episiotomies can often cause serious medical complications. In one recent study, for instance, 6 percent of women given episiotomies suffered from persistent, long-term pain during intercourse. One further effect to note: the incision and stitches from an episiotomy often take a good deal longer to heal than a doctor tells a mother (if he tells at all), and infection and blood loss are common reactions. In the *American Journal of Obstetrics and Gynecology,* P. Shiono et al., reports that episiotomies are likely to produce massive lacerations. These often result in excessive blood loss, painful scarring, and unnecessary postpartum pain in birthing mothers.[36] Christiane Northrup concurs:

> Women who undergo episiotomy are fifty times *more* likely to suffer from severe lacerations than those who don't have it. The reason for this is that episiotomy cuts frequently extend farther into the vaginal tissues during the delivery. . . . The woman's discomfort may affect her bonding with and nursing of the infant. No long-term benefits have been shown for women who have had episiotomies, although I was repeatedly taught that episiotomy was absolutely necessary to prevent a later prolapse of the uterus and/or excessive laxity of the vagina. . . . Episiotomy is a telling example of how in clinical practice a belief—*"Women's bodies can't give birth healthfully without intervention"*—can actually win out over scientific evidence, which in this case supports not doing an episiotomy.[37]

Cesarean Birth

Last on the list of birth and delivery interventions is the cesarean birth (c-section): the baby is delivered directly from the uterus through a surgical incision made along the mother's abdomen.

So much has been reported in the past years, both in mainstream periodicals and TV specials, on the overuse of this surgical procedure and on, as one medical newscaster called it, the "cesarean epidemic" that it seems redundant to repeat the fact that in 2002 the cesarean birth rate shot up to an all-time high of 26.1 percent—and that women who undergo cesarean births are 16 times more likely to die than women who birth vaginally. Translated into human terms, this means that more than one million mothers now give birth via major abdominal surgery, and that accordingly, these women are put at risk.

We must acknowledge that cesarean birth is, in its own way, a miracle of modern medicine and that over the years this operation has saved the lives of countless infants and mothers alike. It is clear that the operation has its place.

It is also estimated, however, that half to three-quarters of these operations are unnecessary. Explanations as to why so many needless c-sections are performed each year are complex and numerous. Reasons include insurance concerns; threat of malpractice suits; lack of adequate training on the part of physicians who are unwilling to take a wait-and-see attitude during labor; premature panic on the part of mother and doctor alike; and economic incentives for the medical establishment, such as less time spent by the doctor at delivery, increased length of hospital stay, and greater reimbursement by third-party payment.

Another reason, more psychological than economic, is summed up by one mother-to-be, who said, "Spare me the process; just give me the product." In our post-modern times it seems even the process of human birth often ranks efficiency as the number one priority, even when such emphasis makes no sense biologically—or emotionally: just deliver me a baby, doc, in the fastest, easiest way you know how.

It should be made clear that cesarean birth is major abdominal surgery, carrying with it all the risks of such procedures: infection, hemorrhage, healing problems, scarring, increased chances of pneumonia, and many more. Further, should they become pregnant again, women who have undergone a c-section are less likely to have a normal vaginal birth than those who have delivered naturally, and in subsequent pregnancies, both mother and baby are at greater risk for tubal pregnancies and abnormalities of the placenta. We know, further, that women who have a c-section are ten times more likely to lose their uteruses because of hemorrhage, a major cause of death among birthing mothers. Imminent physical risks include damage to bowel function, bladder infection, kidney damage, and respiratory complications, all of which can lead to additional surgeries performed to repair the damage done by the c-section itself.

Practically, with cesarean sections there is little or no labor. As a result, there is a disruption in the hormonal peaks of oxytocin, endorphins, adrenal hormones, and prolactin that perform so many miracles. Babies delivered in this manner are also denied the critical adrenalin surge at the time of birth, which thus places the child at a dramatically increased risk of respiratory compromise and even respiratory failure.[38] Another study tells us that a baby's health and risk of death increase during a c-section.[39] The damage, in other words, does not stop with the mother. Nancy Cohen and Louis Estner write: "It is also important not to forget that the infant is also often greatly affected by the cesarean. For example, the newborn may experience jaundice, fewer quiet and alert periods after birth, iatrogenic (hospital induced) respiratory distress due to maternal hypotension, and neonatal death."[40]

On a psychological and emotional level, the long hours of separation between mother and child following a cesarean section cause the first breastfeeding to be delayed to a greater or lesser degree, depending upon the mother's reactions to the drugs and to post-operative pain. One study shows that the 80 percent of women who give birth naturally experience elevation in mood and self-esteem after delivery, compared to the roughly 17 percent who have cesarean sections (and who indeed often suffer from postpartum depression). Incidentally, the balance of the women, 3 percent in this study, had their children delivered by forceps or with vacuum assistance.[41]

Still another study shows that after a cesarean birth, the manufacture of the breastfeeding hormone prolactin is diminished and oxytocin levels in both mother and child are reduced significantly. Because many studies demonstrate a direct relationship between long-term breastfeeding and factors such as increased intelligence, higher immune function, reduced risk of diabetes, lower obesity potential, and even increased immunity to cancer, the absence of breastfeeding in children due to c-section is clearly a detriment to both mother and child.

The good news: There are several ways to minimize the risk of c-section in a normal, low-risk birth:

❧ Make a birth plan ahead of time with the people delivering your baby, letting them know that unless the birth situation is life threatening you prefer to bypass the c-section option.

❧ Avoid epidurals and the drug Pitocin (synthetic oxytocin) to speed up birth. Both increase the need for abdominal delivery. Make it clear ahead of time to those delivering your child that you forbid the use of both of these interventions.

❧ Avoid going to the hospital too early. Statistically, premature hospitalization increases the chances of a mother receiving a c-section.

❧ Use a midwife and, if you choose, a doula. The use of midwives and labor assistants is known to lower c-sections rates. These women are also your educated advocates, providing as natural a childbirth as is possible in your situation.

❧ Avail yourself of the many natural birth techniques outlined in this chapter. All are designed specifically to relax mothers, reduce pain and fear levels, make labor less difficult, and increase the chances of a delivery without complications.

AFTER BIRTH: CUTTING THE UMBILICAL CORD

Dr. William F. Windle studied childbirth practices in hospital deliveries and focused on the practice of cutting the umbilical cord at the moment of birth. He performed a study on monkeys, severing the umbilical cord immediately after birth, as is done in many hospitals today. Interestingly, all the newborn monkeys Windle treated in this way ended up gasping for air and needed to be resuscitated.

Windle then performed autopsies on infant monkeys that died of asphyxiation at birth and found a type of lesion in their brains that results specifically from oxygen deprivation. He was also able to keep alive some half-suffocated monkeys until they reached maturity, at which time he autopsied these animals and found that their brains showed the same type of lesions.

He concluded that the damage done at birth was irreparable. He also extrapolated that cutting the umbilical cord prematurely can have the same effect on children. He likewise theorized from this that the standard method of making a child take its first breath is in reality a process of emergency resuscitation. It is interesting that the universal picture of childbirth is often that of spanking the newborn: holding it upside down and slapping its bottom to bring air into its tired drugged system. Yet nowhere in nature do we see a failure to breathe except in stillborns—and nowhere in the world do we find this emergency measure taken except in modern Western hospitals.

In his book *Magical Child*, Joseph Chilton Pearce reports that Newall Kephart, director of the Achievement Center for Children at Purdue University, found learning and behavioral problems resulting from minor undetected brain injury in 15 to 20 percent of all children who experienced premature cutting of their umbilical cords when they were newborns. Writes Pearce:

> Windle closed his report published in *Scientific America* with this comment: "Our experiments have taught us that birth asphyxia lasting long enough to make resuscitation necessary always damages the brain. . . . A great many human infants have to be resuscitated at birth. We assume that their brains too have been damaged. There is reason to believe that the number of human beings in the United States with minimal brain damage due to asphyxia at birth is much larger than has been thought. Perhaps it is time to reexamine the current practices of childbirth with a view to avoiding conditions that give rise to asphyxia."[42]

In 1801, Erasmus Darwin, grandfather of the famous naturalist Charles Darwin, wrote the following words of advice in his medical textbook: "Another thing very injurious to the child is the tying and cutting of the navel string too soon; which should always be left till the child has not only fully repeatedly breathed, but till all pulsation in the cord ceases. As otherwise the child is much weaker than it ought to be, a portion of the blood being left in the placenta, which ought to have been in the child."[43]

Now we can move the hands of the clock ahead several centuries, to the year 1998. In an article written for a popular obstetric journal, G. M. Morley advises this: "To avoid injury in all deliveries, especially those of neonates at risk, the cord should not be clamped until placental transfusion [the movement of blood from the placenta into the child through the umbilical cord] is complete."[44]

In the two hundred years that have elapsed between these similar medical caveats, literally hundreds of medical textbooks have been published providing the same opinion: the umbilical cord should not be cut until it stops pulsing, a period of time that can run from five to twenty minutes. Indeed, today an entire website is devoted to quotes taken from medical texts and journals dating from the late eighteenth century to the present time warning doctors against this potentially dangerous practice.[45] Here are a few examples:

> From 1981: Immediate cord clamping before the child has breathed should be avoided . . . in certain unfavorable conditions the consequences may be fatal.[46]
>
> From 1982: Immediate cord clamping can result in hypotension, hypovolemia, and anemia.[47]
>
> From 1993: [Delayed clamping, as opposed to immediate clamping,] has clinical and economic benefits.[48]

All other mammals sever the cord only after the placenta is delivered, and, to my knowledge, all traditional cultures follow this practice also. The late severance is safe and ensures that the baby gets an optimal placental transfusion, and that the mother is protected from retained placenta, postpartum hemorrhage, and leakage of the baby's blood into her own circulation.[49]

This last warning is not only recommended in a majority of medical texts, but is also taught in most medical schools today, where a majority of medical lecturers continue to caution students against immediate cord-cutting risks, knowing that early clamping deprives the child of from 54 to 150 ml of vitally needed blood.[50] The physicians who defend early cord clamping insist that waiting too long to clamp the cord floods the newborn with an overabundance of blood, a potentially dangerous condition known as *hypervolemia*. They advocate "active management of the third stage," which means quick severance of the cord accompanied by injections of artificial oxytocin to make the uterus contract, thus bringing the birth process to a conveniently swift close.

Indeed, great haste in clamping is required after these injections because artificially injected oxytocin generates such powerful contractions that the placenta can at times become hopelessly lodged in the uterus, necessitating a surgical operation for its removal. Yet, interestingly, in 1995 the American College of Obstetrics and Gynecology rewrote certain educational bulletins on this subject, eliminating all opposition to immediate cord clamping, presumably because physicians found early clamping to be a harmless and potentially useful tool.

Perhaps—but at the same time, as one doctor points out, neonatal intensive care units are "filled with weak, fast-clamped newborns exhibiting signs of severe blood loss, pallor, low blood volume, anemia, low blood pressure, hypothermia, poor urine output, metabolic acidosis, low oxygen supply, and respiratory distresses to the point that some need blood transfusions, and many more receive blood volume expanders."[51]

The abiding riddle, then, is why so many obstetricians in so many hospitals—physicians who are well educated in the dangers of early clamping and who have been warned by reams of documented evidence and well advised by instructors in their own profession—continue to cut and clamp a newborn's umbilical cord the moment it emerges from the womb.

Important to note here is that before delivery, the mother's placenta provides all the oxygen an unborn child requires to maintain healthy cellular tissue, using the umbilical cord as a conduit. At the moment of birth, the situation changes dramatically: Neonates are forced to adapt from an in-utero water environment, in which oxygen supply and other nourishment are provided copiously, to an open-air environment in which the lungs must quickly take over the job of breathing. During these critical moments of transition, oxygen continues to flow from the placenta into the child via the umbilical cord. As long as this cord continues pulsating, blood and oxygen is being transfused to the child. The moment this transfusion from placenta to child does its job and the child begins to breathe, the vessels in the umbilical cord clamp shut automatically. The pulsations in the cord then subside, and within minutes the cord ceases all activity. At this point it is safe to cut the cord.

So what happens if the umbilical cord is cut and clamped too early—if it is severed and the infant's lungs are still not functioning? In many cases, nothing happens. Though a cord may be snipped prematurely, meaning that all oxygen flow through it is brought to a halt, the newborn is usually able to weather this storm until the crying reflex (or a hard smack on the bottom) shocks its lungs into activity. Certainly, it can never be said that every case of premature clamping causes brain damage.

At the same time, the premature cutting of the cord and the consequent reduction of oxygen flow to the child's brain that results (sometimes for many minutes) can and often does produce serious oxygen deprivation—*hypoxia,* as it is termed in medical usage. Immediate clamping, moreover, forces the baby to switch from a water environment to an air environment in a matter of moments. Many researchers feel that this sudden shift is forced on the child too abruptly, provoking feelings of fear and panic, which in turn reduce oxygen levels further. The condition is made even worse if infants are born under the influence of anesthesia and their systems are working sluggishly. The hypoxia that then follows has been shown in many cases to etch lesions on the brain (as it did in Windle's monkeys and as he suspected that it did in humans). These reduce the child's future intelligence and, many researchers are coming to believe, may be one of the unrecognized contributors to future learning disorders.

In a natural birth, on the other hand, the umbilical cord is allowed to pulse until a newborn breathes on its own gently, slowly, and as a matter of course. Because an infant does not feel choked and because the air is cold on its nubile lungs, it soon begins breathing naturally, regulating the inflow and outflow of air according to its organic needs, just as their inner thermostats dictate. Nature, in short, has designed the process—respiration—to begin organically, on its own, without strangulation, hypoxia, or medical intervention.

Dr. George M. Morley has made a detailed study of the risks involved in early umbilical clamping. He presents some of his most significant findings in the essay "How the Cord Clamp Injures Your Baby's Birth" (footnote 51). According to Morley, an intimidating list of possible side effects may result from premature cutting of the cord:

❧ **Mental deficiency.** When the umbilical cord is allowed to cycle unhindered through the post-birth transfer, delivering a full placental transfusion of blood, enough iron is infused into the child's bloodstream to prevent it from developing anemia for at least the first year of life.

As we know, early anemia—that is, lack of an adequate number of red blood cells in the bloodstream—is a major cause of retardation and mental deficiency in children. Because prematurely clamped infants lack up to one half their normal blood volume, statistically, infant anemia has a greater than average chance of developing in early clamped newborns. This iron deficiency, in turn, can cause mild to severe retardation, learning problems, and a wide variety of behavioral disorders.

❧ **Respiratory distress syndrome (RDS).** This lung disorder impairs breathing, eventually producing a life-threatening lack of oxygen in the blood. In infants, and especially in premature babies, RDS is generated by low volumes of oxygen-rich blood entering the lungs.

For many years, an overwhelming amount of evidence has pointed to the fact that early cord clamping produces RDS in neonates. In one experiment, a doctor prevented this condition in newborns simply by suspending the placenta and cord over the infant like an intravenous drip, allowing the force of gravity to do its work and to keep the child fully transfused and oxygenated until its lungs started working on their own.[52]

✤ **Brain hemorrhage.** Brain hemorrhage, or intraventricular hemorrhage (IVA), is often associated with respiratory distress syndrome in premature babies. When it is deprived of sufficient oxygen by early clamping, premature infant's brain tissue dies quickly and hemorrhage occurs into the dead tissue and parts of the brain. Writes Morley, "Later, absorption of dead tissue enlarges the ventricle. These preemies have permanent neurological defects. No studies allowing preemies to close their own umbilical cords and to achieve normal blood volumes have ever been done."[53]

✤ **Cerebral palsy.** When a child is born with its umbilical cord wrapped around its neck, it almost always undergoes severe oxygen deprivation. If such a depressed infant is resuscitated by keeping the cord and placenta in place and pumping blood while the lungs are ventilated, it has a good chance of recovery—but if the infant's umbilical cord is cut abruptly, depriving it of placental blood, the newborn is even more deprived of oxygen and severe hypoxic brain damage can result. Many studies show that in the months that follow, this damage may produce the motor reflexes symptomatic of cerebral palsy.

Morley's article continues in this vein, giving solid medical evidence as to how premature clamping leads to such conditions as colitis, hyaline membrane disease,[54] and other serious medical complications. His studies take their place along hundreds like them, all asking that doctors allow at least a few minutes to elapse before cutting the umbilical cord to allow it and the placenta to do the work nature intended.

In natural childbirth, this method is practiced as a matter of course. For parents practicing conventional delivery, options are still open. One scenario: simply let your obstetrician know before the delivery that you have strong feelings concerning early clamping and that you prefer that the cord remain uncut until it stops pulsing and the child begins breathing of its own volition. Most responsible physicians will oblige.

In our birth experience when Dalit pushed sufficiently so that

Kesem's head and little shoulders came out, I reached down and took him under the arms and lifted him out and picked him up and held his little wet body close to the towel I had draped across me. I held him away from me with the umbilical cord still attached and looked straight into his eyes, which were wide open and staring back at me. He had started breathing on his own and I put him down, skin to skin, on Dalit's belly. After the cord stopped throbbing, I cut the cord and the midwife tied it off.

APPROACHING THE FOURTH TRIMESTER

By using the many natural birth options explained in this chapter and avoiding the medical interventions and techniques that are so likely to confuse nature's organic birthing road map, a newborn is brought from the womb and into the world in a blaze of awe, ecstasy, and joy. Life has begun.

From the perspective of natural childbirth, however, with this entrance, the process of birth is only partially complete. What takes place next is connected intimately to the moment of your child's delivery—it is a continuation of it, really—and to the assurance of a healthy baby. In the chapters that follow, we will explore how and why a scientifically based natural birth requires a number of additional actions on the part of parents during the first hours, days, and weeks following delivery if a child's birth is to achieve its full potential. This includes the all-important act of breastfeeding. The new parenting refers to this critical post-birth period as "the fourth trimester."

The actions that follow birth—so critical to the quality of a newborn's health and mental growth—are demanding to some extent and taxing in a number of ways, but at the same time, they are gloriously rewarding. For some parents they produce moments of delight and euphoria that approach the elation inspired by the birth itself.

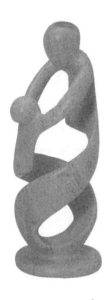

5

Breastfeeding

*If a multinational company developed a product that was
a nutritionally balanced and delicious food, a wonder
drug that both prevented and treated disease, cost almost
nothing to produce and could be delivered in quantities
controlled by the consumers' needs, the very announcement
of their find would send their shares rocketing to the
top of the stock market. The scientists who developed the
product would win prizes, and the wealth and influence
of everyone involved would increase dramatically. Women
have been producing such a miraculous substance, breast
milk, since the beginning of human existence.*

GABRIELLE PALMER

IN THIS CHAPTER YOU will not learn how to breastfeed. There is
already plenty of solid advice in this area from a number of authoritative sources, including natural baby-care professionals, Internet
Web sites, prebirth training classes, magazines and books written
on childcare, friends and relatives who have already gone the breastfeeding route, institutions such as La Leche League that specialize
in disseminating breastfeeding information, and doctors and nurses
who are friendly to new parenting techniques. These and many other

sources can advise, instruct, and train you in the principles of nursing your child.

Instead of focusing on how, here I first ask you to take a step back, to the period of time before a child is born—the time when parents-to-be are making crucial decisions: Should we pursue natural childbirth or conventional birth? Which obstetrician should we choose? Which hospital or birthing center should we choose? Should we get a sonogram (ultrasound)? And perhaps the most pointed question of all once the child is born: should we breastfeed our child?

Included here is information on *why* you should breastfeed—and why breastfeeding goes such a long way in improving and protecting the life of a child and the life of a mother.

What you won't find here: the scare tactics that are too frequently the centerpiece of books and articles on nursing. The social, psychological, and scientific facts of breastfeeding are sufficiently persuasive and compelling without such a gloss. All you must do: read this chapter carefully, weigh the pros and cons presented, and then decide for yourself whether home nursing is right for you and your child.

THE EXPERTS SPEAK

In 1996 the American Academy of Pediatrics summarized its position on breastfeeding: "The benefits of breastfeeding are so numerous that the Academy strongly encourages the practice during the first six to twelve months of life. Human milk is nutritionally superior to formulas for the content of fats, cholesterol, and proteins; all substitute-feeding options differ markedly from it. There is evidence that human milk confers protection against infection from other diseases."

In explaining the many ways in which breastfeeding improves the interaction between mother and child, Dr. William Sears, doyen of natural pediatric wisdom in the United States, tells us this:

Breastfeeding mothers respond to their babies more intuitively and with less restraint. The baby's signals of hunger or distress trigger a biological response in the mother (a milk letdown), and she feels the urge to pick up the baby and nurse him. This responsiveness rewards both mother and baby with good feelings. If a mother is bottle-feeding, her response to her baby's hunger or distress cues is quite different. She must initially divert her attention away from the baby to an object, the bottle, and take time to find and prepare it. Research has shown that a baby's memory span in the first six months is from four to ten seconds. The time it takes to produce a nonbiological response, such as bottle-feeding, is usually longer than the baby's memory span. The bottle-feeding baby does not receive the same immediate reinforcement of his cues that a breastfeeding baby does. In my practice, I have noticed that breastfeeding mothers tend to show a higher degree of sensitivity to their babies, and I believe this is a result of the biological changes that occur in a mother in response to the signals of her child.[1]

This statement is from the World Health Organization (WHO), currently a staunch supporter of breastfeeding and proper childhood nutrition:

Breastfeeding is an unequalled way of providing ideal food for the healthy growth and development of infants; it is also an integral part of the reproductive process with important implications for the health of mothers. A recent review of evidence has shown that, on a population basis, exclusive breastfeeding for six months is the optimal way of feeding infants. Thereafter infants should receive complementary foods with continued breastfeeding up to two years of age or beyond.[2]

To enable mothers to establish and sustain exclusive breastfeeding for six months, WHO and UNICEF recommend:

- Initiation of breastfeeding within the first hour of life
- Exclusive breastfeeding—that is, the infant receives only breast milk without any additional food or drink, not even water
- Breastfeeding on demand—that is, as often as the child wants, day and night
- No use of bottles, teats, or pacifiers

The WHO goes on to say:

> Breast milk is the natural first food for babies, it provides all the energy and nutrients that the infant needs for the first months of life, and it continues to provide up to half or more of a child's nutritional needs during the second half of the first year, and up to one-third during the second year of life.
>
> Breast milk promotes sensory and cognitive development, and protects the infant against infectious and chronic diseases. Exclusive breastfeeding reduces infant mortality due to common childhood illnesses such as diarrhea or pneumonia, and helps for a quicker recovery during illness. . . . Breastfeeding contributes to the health and well-being of mothers, it helps to space children, reduces the risk of ovarian cancer and breast cancer, increases family and national resources, is a secure way of feeding, and is safe for the environment.[3]

Dr. Miriam Labbok, UNICEF's senior advisor for infant and young child feeding and care, adds this about the virtues of breast milk and the drawbacks of formula:

> First, formula, at its best, only replaces most nutritional components of breast milk. Breast milk changes with the time of the day, the duration of suckling and the age of the child. In addition, breast milk carries passive factors that fight disease, and when breastfed, the infant gets active living cells from the mother that help combat disease.

Further, in the first few months, it is hard for the baby's gut to absorb foreign substances. If you give even one feeding of formula or other foods, you may be causing micro-injuries to the gut and it takes weeks for the baby to recover. In any case, you will disrupt the living cells and normal bacteria that inhabit the gut and support digestion. The act of breastfeeding itself stimulates proper growth of the mouth and jaw, and secretion of hormones for digestion and satiety.

Finally, there are hundreds of other factors in breast milk that you cannot include in formula—everything from bifudus factor, which helps the gut grow, and long chain fatty acids that help the brain grow, to hormones and enzymes that aid development. Studies have shown that breastfed infants do better on intelligence and behavior tests into adulthood. There has never been a study that shows any advantage of formula feeding over breastfeeding.[4]

THE BIG NO-BRAINER

Thousands, or more realistically, many thousands of authoritative statements from renowned doctors and institutions around the world could be cited in place of the preceding quotes. All have one thing in common: They stress the positive emotional impact of breastfeeding on mother and child alike and its nutritional superiority over bottle-feeding.

These expert voices not only recommend breastfeeding; they urge it. They contend that by denying newborns this natural and multisided support, parents deprive them forever of profound advantages that innumerable studies now show make infants happier, smarter, calmer, and healthier human beings.

Yet despite so many urgings from so many world-renowned experts, many physicians, and hence many new mothers, still look on breast-feeding with a raised eyebrow. Studies evaluating the factors that cause American women to say no to this ancient maternal option reveal a sizeable list of obstacles. Primary among them are lack of support from family, friends, spouse, and society; insufficient prenatal breastfeeding education from obstetricians and hospitals; fear of discomfort; lack of time at home; and, of course, media pressures that drum into public consciousness the supposed nutritional superiority of commercial formula over mother's milk.[5]

The good news is that despite its many opponents, breastfeeding is increasing at a steady rate in the United States. Efforts made by certain baby-friendly doctors and hospitals are resulting in improved post-birth education, and more than ever before, mothers are opting for mother's milk over formula.

At the same time, the truth is that many mothers in this country do not nurse and that the present status quo throws many thorns in their path if they choose to pursue breastfeeding. On average, a mother who opts to home nurse leaves the hospital within forty-eight hours after her baby is delivered. Up to this time, typically, she receives little or no advice from doctors or hospital personnel on the mechanics of when, where, why, and how to breastfeed her newborn. In some cases family obstetricians make it emphatically clear that they oppose this option entirely and that they urge the new mother to take the "safer," more conventional bottle-feeding route.

Meanwhile, the new mother, already worried by such warnings, arrives home and starts to breastfeed without any information on how to deal with the difficulties that sometimes occur in the course of nursing: sore nipples, infant weight loss, clogged milk ducts, and the like. One study found that 72 percent of new mothers have questions concerning breastfeeding technique during the first few weeks after birth, the time in which most nursing problems occur. In many instances these questions go unresolved.

Because a large number of women in this country did not breastfeed from the 1940s through the 1980s, many new mothers receive little encouragement at home from mothers and grandmothers. Senior generations often look on breastfeeding, as one client of mine describes her mother's words, as "a hippie thing." As recently as 2006 a woman filed a complaint against a commercial airline because she had been asked to exit the airplane when she refused to stop breastfeeding her child. Because family elders were sold a bill of goods by baby-food manufacturers when they did their own parenting, these "advisers" often insist that infants are better nourished with "scientifically balanced" formula and that prolonged breastfeeding can lead to infant malnutrition and serious medical problems for both mother and child. Many fathers, equally untutored in the subtleties of breastfeeding, are all too ready to cave in to these prejudices.

Not knowing where to turn, a new breastfeeding mother consults books, the most common source for breastfeeding information in this country, but all too often her questions go unanswered. Friends know little on the subject, and some are opposed to the whole idea of home nursing. Finally, frazzled by the rigors of the delivery and by lack of sleep and unable to deal with an abscessed nipple or a child who refuses to take the breast, new moms turn to bottle feeding out of sheer desperation simply because no one has told them beforehand that the problems they are facing are common and easily solvable.

There are many other perceived deterrents to breastfeeding standing in the way of eager mothers who simply wish to suckle their newborn babes in the way that infants have been nursed since the time of Eve. Yet rather than recount a laundry list of these objections here, it seems best simply to allow the many scientific and emotional facts of human lactation to speak for themselves. Once most pregnant and aspiring mothers hear the evidence for breastfeeding, even in the thumbnail way that space here allows, this information becomes overwhelming and the verdict becomes a no-brainer: Most women who are educated in the subject agree enthusiastically that breastfeeding is clearly and unequivocally the superior way to nourish a child, a mother—and the world.

On a personal note, as I watched my wife, Dalit, nursing our son, Kesem, over the years, it was difficult for me to understand how a new mother would want to miss this exquisite opportunity to connect with and nurture her newborn in the most joyous, intimate, and satisfying way known to mammalian creatures, especially humans, throughout time.

With this in mind, though, we must be aware that each set of parents has its own special needs and priorities. Readers can remember this as they read on, and mothers must remember that the choice is theirs.

THE BENEFITS OF BREASTFEEDING

We know that breastfeeding benefits both the mother and the child. Outlined here are the positive impacts on each participant and on the family as a whole.

Benefits to the Child

Many parents-to-be know that nursing increases the bond between mother and child, that it exerts some type of birth control, and that there are nutrients in mother's milk that help promote and protect an infant's health. Usually, however, this knowledge is sketchy and incomplete. Other than experts in the field of lactation or those who have researched the subject thoroughly, most of us remain unaware of the surprising and sometimes astonishing effects that mother's milk, delivered warm and delicious to the palette of the hungry child, can provide. Here are some of these benefits, which, in many cases, stem from findings of the last decade.

Breastfeeding boosts your child's intelligence level. According to a study of one thousand infants performed at the Christchurch School of Medicine in New Zealand,[6] infants who are breastfed for eight months not only have higher IQs than formula-fed children, but also, when school days roll around, they demonstrate increased problem-solving ability in class, have superior reading comprehension, develop better math skills, and gain higher grades.

Another 1999 study reports that an analysis of twenty studies on breastfeeding and brain development shows that as breastfed children mature in the first months following birth, their intelligence level is five IQ points higher than children who are bottle-fed. Babies who are breastfed for up to six months demonstrate the greatest increase in IQ, while children breastfed for less than two weeks show no improvement at all. According to analysis, the actual bonding of a mother and child, with its associated affections and pleasures—which are like food to an infant, is responsible for 40 percent of this increase in brainpower. The remaining 60 percent is due to nutrients in the milk itself.[7]

Two of the key ingredients in human milk are DHA and ARA. Members of the much-touted omega-3 fatty acid family, both play a central role in early brain-tissue growth and development and hence in infant intelligence gains. Significantly, autopsies of infants reveal that milk-fed babies have higher concentrations of both DHA and ARA in their brain tissue than formula-fed babies.

Studies also show that children who are breastfed have better sight than nonbreastfed babies—probably, scientists think, because of these same crucial fats in the milk. Yet while mother's milk is full of both these enriching substances, they are absent entirely from every commercial brand of baby formula on the market.

Here, it should also be mentioned that other fats in breast milk (though not found in formula), specifically linoleic and linolenic fatty acids, help develop the healthy growth of *myelin,* a lipid and protein substance that forms a protective sheath around certain nerve fibers, especially those found on the spine. (Eroded myelin spots on the spine can cause multiple sclerosis.)

Proteins also play a role in the development of the brain. As we know, they are the primary building blocks of the human mass. Though mother's milk does not contain vast amounts of proteins—an overload at a very early age can stress a child's system—it does contain generous amounts of the protein taurine, an amino acid that plays an integral part in early development of brain and eye cells. Because the body is incapable of converting other types of amino acids into taurine, mother's milk provides this needed food directly from the breast. Interestingly, because it is now an established fact that taurine plays a critical part in nerve growth and we understand that a lack of it impedes early brain development, some baby food manufacturers are at last adding synthetic forms of it to their formula.

Another important growth ingredient delivered directly from human milk is the nutrient choline, a vitamin-like substance related to the B-family. Once in the bloodstream choline helps manufacture acetylcholine, a principal neurotransmitter in the brain that aids us in thinking, acting, and functioning. One study at the University of North Carolina reveals that without sufficient levels of choline in an infant's body, nerve cells divide less and multiply less, impeding the maturity of the brain and nervous system.[8] Most commercial formulas contain no choline.

Sugar—especially lactose, the main sugar in mother's milk—also plays a fundamental part in early development of human intelligence. Once broken down in the liver, lactose is turned into two simple sugars: galactose and glucose. Both are vital nutrients for developing brain matter. Store-bought formula contains no lactose and is filled instead with refined cane sugar, one of the least nourishing and, some would say, one of the most harmful of all substances in the food kingdom.

Another major builder of childhood brain cells is cholesterol. Given a bad name by doctors and dieticians, this fatty lipid produces vital hormones and bile salts in a child's system and plays a major part in transporting nutritious fats to hungry cell tissues via the bloodstream. Cholesterol also helps the growth of new nerve cells in the brain. Breast milk is loaded with cholesterol, but commercial formula contains none.[9]

Breastfeeding may help reduce your child's chances of developing heart problems as an adult. Medical researchers now know that breast milk contains a number of long-chain polyunsaturated fatty acids. These acids insure the healthy growth of an infant's coronary system. They also prevent heart problems from occurring during the first weeks of life.

In one project at the Institute of Child Health in England,[10] 926 babies were studied in order to determine the relationship between breastfeeding and healthy hearts. Some of these infants were assigned to receive breast milk; others were scheduled to receive formula. Sixteen years later, researchers were able to track down 216 of these young subjects and study their blood for markers of heart health and cholesterol levels, including "bad" (HDL, or high-density lipoprotein) levels, "good" (LDL, or low-density lipoprotein) levels, certain proteins, and other telling signs. Their findings showed that breastfed children displayed markedly lower ratios of HDL to LDL than bottle-fed control-group subjects. Breastfed subjects also had lower blood concentrations of CRP, a protein known to encourage atherosclerosis.

One of the participating doctors in this study, Dr. A. Singhai, went on record as saying that breastfeeding also reduces infant risk of high blood pressure, obesity, and cardiovascular disease. Dr. Singhai claims that the "relative overnutrition" provided by formula feeding can alter a child's metabolism and lead to significant cardiovascular risks in adult life.

Finally, another study warns of another kind of infant heart peril: according to the work of doctors J. Koenig, A. Davies, and B. Thach,[11] during feeding, infants who are bottle-fed are at increased risk of developing cardiopulmonary disturbances, including prolonged airway closure and obstructed respiratory breathing due to repeated swallowing.

Breastfeeding can make your child's immune system bulletproof. Human milk offers newborns a variety of powerful immunoglobulins, or antibodies. These microscopic immune-system soldiers provide protection against the all-too-common ailments to which infants are prone in the first few months of life: colic, diarrhea, colds, digestion problems, and allergies. Innumerable studies show that children who breastfeed have an increased ability to fight off the bacteria and viruses that cause these disorders.

The highest concentration of infant-system antibodies is found in a substance known as *colostrum,* a thick, yellowish fluid produced in the fatty tissue of the breasts during late pregnancy and in the first few days after childbirth. Writes Joseph Chilton Pearce:

> The first milk (colostrum) transfers to the infant the mother's immunities gained over her lifetime. This first milk may contain a hormone that counteracts any excess adrenals to bring the infant's system back into hormonal balance, and further, nursing activates the mandibular joint of the jaw, which is connected to the vestibular rotation factor of the inner ear, which, in turn, is vital to body balance and to orientation of sounds in space.[12]

Replaced by mature breast milk about a week after birth, pure colostrum also contains a mother lode of minerals and proteins, especially secretory IGA, an antibody that attaches itself to the lining of the nose and throat and protects the child against infection in the nose, mouth, and digestive tract. If a newborn does not receive this precious elixir during the first week of birth, statistically, it has a considerably higher chance of acquiring these ailments.[13] A study by the American Academy of Pediatrics shows that: "In evaluating the benefits of breast milk, there is strong evidence to show that breast milk lowers the occurrence and perhaps the seriousness of a number of diseases including urinary tract infections, diarrhea, lower respiratory infections, and bacterial meningitis." Other studies show a decrease in *non-infectious* diseases such as eczema and asthma.[14]

The list of immunological benefits that breast milk delivers is lengthy and growing constantly. Here, for example, are other substances in mother's milk that help improve a baby's line of defense against disease:

§ **Lactoferrin.** Found primarily in colostrum, this is a kind of intestinal gatekeeper, deciding which bacteria can enter and which must die. In the gut it acts as an invincible antibiotic on common harmful bacteria such as strep and *E. coli*.

* **Carnitine.** This vitamin-like compound helps transform fats in a child's system into a source of energy and cell growth. Breastfed babies have a good deal more carnitine in their bloodstreams than bottle-fed babies.

* **Lysozyme.** This is an antibacterial enzyme present in many body fluids such as tears, sweat, and saliva. Human breast milk is rich in this natural antibiotic, which helps destroy a number of potentially harmful microorganisms.

* **Lactobacillaceae.** Various substances in human milk nurture the growth of helpful intestinal microorganisms—lactobacillaceae, which aid digestion and serve as a line of defense against bacterial infection and parasites. Breastfed babies have approximately ten times more of these friendly bacteria in their intestinal tracts than non-breastfed infants.

* **White blood cells.** Human milk is rich in living white blood cells. This means that every time an infant nurses at the breast, it receives millions of these life-sustaining, disease-fighting organisms. Bottle formula contains nothing comparable.

* **Vitamins and minerals.** Mother's milk is a cornucopia of vitamins and minerals, many—perhaps most—of which commercial formula lacks or contains in lab-synthesized versions. At each breastfeeding, large portions of zinc, calcium, selenium, and iron pour into the infant, enriching its blood and making its immunological systems stronger.

Breastfeeding can prevent both common and deadly diseases in your child. Because the many nourishing substances in human milk build powerful defense systems in a child's body, he or she is able to fend off many crippling and some killing diseases—but only if a child breastfeeds for at least several months. Here is a sampling:

❖ **Ear infections.** As we have learned, human milk contains antibodies that produce an antibiotic effect on infection, pouncing on invading germs and dissolving them quickly. As a rule, infants are prone to upper respiratory ailments such as colds and runny noses. These problems cause the middle ear to fill with fluids, which can easily become infected, causing fever, malaise, and the terrible pain of earache. The antibiotic ingredients in breast milk provide a strong line of protection against these unpleasant episodes.

In addition, the incidence of ear infection is affected by an infant's position while feeding. Writes Dr. Sears, "Because breastfed babies are fed in a more upright position, they're less likely to experience milk backing up through the Eustachian tubes into their ears; if this does happen during a breastfeeding session, human milk is less irritating to the tissues of the middle ear than is formula."[15]

✦ **Obesity.** Researchers at Cincinnati Children's Hospital recently conducted a study of a mother's milk protein known as adiponectin. Many of them believe the presence of this substance in human milk explains the association between breastfeeding and the apparent reduced risk of obesity in adults. Adiponectin is manufactured by fat cells and helps control the way in which the body assimilates sugars and lipids in the bloodstream. High levels of adiponectin are associated with less disease and a more stable weight.

If adiponectin levels are high in human milk, the Cincinnati researchers also theorized, this protein might well influence the metabolic programming of infants, helping them to keep their weight at an even keel and prevent obesity, both during childhood and later on as grownups. Researchers studied samples of human milk and found that, indeed, adiponectin levels are "quite high in human milk—higher than many proteins found in human milk." In milk samples they also discovered the presence of leptin, a protein that plays a significant role in regulation of body fat.[16]

Another study carried out at the same institution reveals "human milk protects extremely low birth-weight babies from developing sepsis—an overwhelming infection, and a leading cause of illness and death in tiny babies. In fact, the more human milk given as a percentage of nutritional intake, the lower the risks of sepsis during the hospital stay." The Cincinnati Children's researchers analyzed data from 1,270 infants enrolled in another unrelated study carried out at fifteen different medical centers. Thirty-nine percent of the infants in these studies suffered from sepsis infection. Significantly, this group also received a good deal less human milk than infants who remained healthy.

❖ **Strong, well-aligned teeth.** Studies show that when children nurse for at least six months, the sucking action and the position of the mouth on the breast help the tongue and facial muscles to assume optimum alignment, preventing problems such as overbite and a poorly aligned jaw. A study of ten thousand children showed that infants who were breastfed had a 40 percent lower need for orthodontia in their teenage years than children raised on the bottle.[17]

Meanwhile, a study at the University of Athens in Greece gives evidence that nursing helps prevent tooth decay. Scientists studied 260 children between the ages of three and five. These children were divided into two groups: those with many cavities and those with few. It was determined that children who were breastfed for more than forty days after birth were considerably less likely to develop cavities than those who were breastfed for shorter periods of time or not at all. Infants at highest risk for developing tooth decay were those who fell asleep with a bottle in their mouths. A separate study published in *Pediatric Dentistry* in 1999 concluded that human breast milk is not cariogenic—that is, it does not cause cavities.[18]

❖ **Lower risk of infant mortality in the first year.** At the National Institute of Environmental Health Services, information gathered from several studies suggests that breastfeeding reduces the risk of death for infants in their first year. In one study, researchers compared Center for Disease Control (CDC) records of 1,204 children who died between twenty-eight days of life and one year with 7,740 children who were alive and healthy after this period of time. As it turns out, breastfed children have a 20 percent lower risk of dying in their first year of life than children who are bottle-fed. The longer the period of time a child is breastfed, the less likely he or she is to die from both chronic and acute disorders.[19]

✤ **Protection against Sudden Infant Death Syndrome (SIDS).** According to the Association of SIDS and Infant Mortality Programs (ASIP), several studies have found SIDS to be less common in breast-fed infants than in children who take formula. The association reports that a study in New Zealand discovered that nursing has "a significant association with lowered SIDS risk when exclusive breastfeeding was continued during the first six months of life." ASIP does, however, add that, "Research of the relationship of SIDS and infant feeding has been marred by methodological problems, including insufficient sample size and inadequate definition of breastfeeding."[20]

Another study, this one carried out in Scandinavia in 2002, compared 244 babies who died of SIDS with 869 healthy babies. They discovered that babies who were breastfed for four months or more have a considerably higher chance of avoiding SIDS than those who nurse for eight weeks or less.[21]

Finally, respiratory ailments are considered to be one of the possible causes of SIDS. As we have seen, mother's milk fights infection and thus reduces the number of nose-stopping, airway-clogging colds that may contribute to SIDS. It is also hypothesized by researchers that there are certain substances in mother's milk that may kill as yet unidentified viruses and bacteria that in some way contribute to this heartbreaking disease.

✤ **Help against a host of other diseases.** Though some of the studies on the relationship between nursing and prevention of the following diseases are inconclusive or require further research, there is much evidence that breastfeeding does, in fact, provide babies—and later, adults—with a degree of protection against the following ailments. The quotes included are taken from studies on the diseases mentioned:

1. **Respiratory allergies and colds.** "Breastfeeding, even for short periods, was clearly associated with lower incidence of wheezing, prolonged colds, diarrhea, and vomiting."[22]

2. **Food allergies.** "Breastfeeding for longer than one month without other milk supplement offers significant prophylaxis against food allergy at three years of age."[23]

3. **Eczema.** "Eczema was less common and milder in babies who were breastfed (22 percent), and whose mothers were on a restricted diet (48 percent). In infants fed casein hydrolysate, soymilk, or cow's milk, 21, 63, and 70 percent, respectively, developed atopic eczema."[24]

4. **Diarrhea.** "Children less than twelve months of age had a lower incidence of acute diarrheal disease during the months they were being breastfed than children who were fed with formula during the same period."[25]

5. **Multiple sclerosis.** "Although thought to be multifactorial in origin, and without a clearly defined etiology, lack of breastfeeding does appear to be associated with an increased incidence of multiple sclerosis."[26]

6. **Colitis.** "Among babies born at more than thirty weeks gestation, confirmed necrotizing enteral colitis was rare in those whose diet included breast milk. It was 20 times more common in those fed formula only."[27]

7. **Diabetes Mellitus.** "Children who developed [diabetes] in New South Wales, Australia, were matched with healthy children (ratio 1:2) of the same sex and age for comparison. Those who were exclusively breastfed during their first three months of life had a 34 percent lower risk of developing diabetes than those who were not breastfed. Children given cow's milk-based formula in their first three months were 52 percent more likely to develop diabetes than those not given cow's milk formula."[28]

8. **Constipation.** "Mother's milk is a natural laxative. It is filled with friendly bacteria that supports infant digestion, and helps prevent diarrhea and constipation."[29]

9. **Bronchitis.** "The authors presented results found in infants

with two or more episodes of acute chronic bronchitis. They found that approximately twice as many bottle-fed infants presented with the problems as those who were breastfed."[30]

10. **Herpes Simplex.** "Mother's milk could play a role in the protection of newborns from Herpes Simplex virus II contamination."[31]

11. **Gastroesophageal Reflex.** "Breastfed neonates demonstrate gastroesophageal reflux episodes of significantly shorter duration than formula-fed neonates."[32]

12. **Hodgkins Disease.** "[There is] a statistically significant protective effect against Hodgkin's disease among children who are breastfed at least eight months, compared with children who were breastfed no more than two months."[33]

13. **Childhood cancer.** "Children who are artificially fed or breastfed for only six months or less are at an increased risk of developing cancer before the age of fifteen. The risk of artificially fed children was 1–9 times that of long-term breastfed children, and the risk for short-term feeders was 1–9 times that of long-term breast feeders."[34]

14. **Crohn's Disease.** "In this study, lack of breastfeeding was a risk factor associated with later development of Crohn's disease."[35]

15. **Type B influenza.** "In a population-based case control study of risk factors for primary invasion of haemophilus influenza, type B disease; breastfeeding was protective of infants less than six months of age."[36]

16. **Juvenile Rheumatoid Arthritis (JRA).** "Preliminary data from researchers at the University of North Carolina and Duke University comparing fifty-four children with JRA and a control group without JRA of similar age and race indicates that children who were breastfed were only 40 percent as likely to develop JRA."[37]

Benefits to the Mother

Writes Alicia Dermer, M.D., a recognized lactation expert and teacher:

> Often, mothers see breastfeeding as martyrdom to be endured for
> their baby's health. If they stop early, they may feel guilty about
> depriving the baby of some health benefits, but their guilt is often
> soothed by well-meaning people who reassure them that "the baby
> will do just as well on formula." Perhaps if they knew that continu-
> ing to breastfeed is also good for their own health, some mothers
> might be less likely to quit when they run into problems. Indeed,
> many mothers are not being told how good breastfeeding is for their
> health. Many health care providers fail to inform mothers of the
> facts. It's time for this well-kept secret to come out.[38]

In short, infants are not the only ones who benefit from breastfeeding. Nature has designed it so that any mother who breastfeeds her offspring will be granted wonderful rewards in return.

**Breastfeeding helps new mothers recover physically from child-
birth more quickly.** Breastfeeding contributes substantially to maternal
health in the weeks following childbirth. This widely recognized benefit
is due to the fact that the mechanism of breastfeeding helps the mother's
uterus contract more rapidly than it would if she was not nursing from
the breast. The effect of these contractions reduces blood loss in the new
mother, lessens the chance of developing infection, and aids in healing.
Many childcare professionals actually consider these uterine contractions, helped along by breastfeeding, to be the final stage of labor.

On a psychological level, a breastfeeding mother tends to feel extremely
positive about herself and her infant. These emotions are inspired not
simply by pride of motherhood. Instead, they are caused by physical stimulation produced by two hormones, which are prevalent in mother's milk
and which we have already discussed: prolactin, which encourages relaxation and affection and which fights stress, and oxytocin, the so-called

love hormone, which helps mothers bond to their children and to just plain feel good about themselves, their life, and the world around them.

Besides producing euphoric states in many nursing mothers, breast-feeding is a specific against post-delivery letdown and, in some cases, postpartum depression. Bottle-feeding commercial baby formula provides neither of these joy-inducing hormones.

Breastfeeding lowers a mother's chances of developing certain types of cancer.

✤ **Breast cancer.** Scientific research has identified certain harmful lifestyle habits and natural conditions that tend to increase a woman's chances of developing breast cancer. Along with factors such as obesity, early menstruation, late menopause, drinking alcohol, smoking, having a close relative with breast cancer, taking hormone replacement therapy, and being over the age of thirty when delivering a first baby, it is known that mothers who breastfeed have approximately a 25 percent lower chance of developing breast cancer than those who bottle-feed their child. It is generally believed that these benefits kick in after the fourth month of nursing at the breast, and breastfeeding for at least six months to a year offers even stronger protection.

✤ **Ovarian cancer.** "Breastfeeding should be added to the list of factors that decrease ovulatory age and thereby decrease the risk of ovarian cancer," writes A. P. Schneider in a study reported in the *New England Journal of Medicine*.[39] To this advice the American Cancer Society adds, "Pregnancy and breastfeeding seem to lower the risk of ovarian cancer, especially when a woman has her first baby before age 30. But choices about when to have a child should not be made just for the purpose of reducing ovarian cancer risk, especially since using birth control pills will have a similar impact."[40]

✤ **Uterine cancer.** According to an Australian study on uterine cancer, women who breastfeed develop this disease less often than women who never nurse at the breast. Writes the authors of the study: "A protective effect against uterine cancer was found for women who breastfeed."[41]

Early breastfeeding stops a woman from becoming pregnant too quickly following birth. One of the major fears mothers have after going through the rigors of pregnancy and childbirth is becoming pregnant again too soon afterward—say, six months after delivery, before they have time to recover from the first birth and to get to know their new infant's habits, ways, and needs.

Happily, nature helps out in this department. During the process of breastfeeding, certain hormones are released into the mother's bloodstream that stop ovulation and hence menses, preventing the release of certain fertility hormones into the blood and shutting down her baby-making potential.

Breastfeeding does work well as a contraceptive—but it is not foolproof. To be certain to avoid pregnancy, new mothers are advised to supplement nature's benefits with their chosen methods of birth control. At the same time, according to a method developed by lactation experts over the past ten years—Lactational Amenorrhea Method (LAM)—if a mother can answer no to the following three questions, she has only a 2 percent chance of becoming pregnant during the early nursing days:

1. Has your monthly cycle returned yet?
2. Do you allow more than three hours in between daytime breastfeedings and six hours in between nighttime breastfeedings?
3. Is your baby older than six months?

To this system, Dr. William Sears adds the following caveats:

§ Practice unrestricted breastfeeding without regard to schedules. Usually six to eight breastfeedings a day will suppress ovulation.

§ Do not train your baby to sleep through the night (the milk-making hormones that suppress ovulation are at their highest between 1 A.M. and 6 A.M.) Nighttime nursing is important to the suppression of fertility. Sleeping with your baby facilitates unrestricted feeding at night.[42]

Breastfeeding mothers gain a measure of protection against osteo-porosis. During lactation, a mother may experience a decrease in bone minerals. Indeed, bone mineral density may be reduced in a mother's body by as much as 1 to 2 percent while she is nursing. This reduction in bone mass, however, is not cause for alarm. After weaning, mothers quickly regain lost bone density, and in the process, the mineral density of their bones often increases, providing post-menopausal protection against osteoporosis. Research also shows that the increase in bone mass formed as a result of breastfeeding may protect women against hip fractures and other types of broken bones in old age. Finally, the overall severity and mortality of rheumatoid arthritis is worse in women who have never breastfed than in those who have.[43]

According to a report put out by La Leche League International on the link between breastfeeding and osteoporosis prevention:

Because calcium is one important element in producing human milk, some health professionals had mistakenly assumed an increased risk of osteoporosis for women who breastfed their children. However, research studies have shown that after weaning their children, breastfeeding mothers' bone density returns to prepregnancy or even higher levels. In one study, researchers examined women who had at least six children each, and who had breastfed for a minimum of six months; these women were compared with women who were never pregnant. Results showed no significant decrease in bone mineral density and no osteoporosis attributable to the multiple pregnancies and extended breastfeeding.[44]

Breastfeeding saves money. A friend and mother named Rosy Allison told me,

One day I sat down and wondered how much money breastfeeding had saved on my grocery bills. I started to do the math. Formula at the supermarket or drug store is expensive and is getting more expensive each year. As any bottle-feeding mom will tell you, babies rip through formula like Grant through Richmond. My girlfriend told me that it seemed to her that she was at the supermarket every five minutes, replenishing the dwindling supplies, then later on stocking up on milk products. Finally, there's the paraphernalia: the bottles, nipples, cups, stuff—all of which seem built to wear out as fast as possible. I figured that by nursing my Jenny, I saved myself and my family around a thousand dollars a year.

Rosy's estimate is nearly accurate. As reported by Dr. Sears, the official statistic is that it costs a family twelve hundred dollars a year to formula-feed one baby.

The American Academy of Pediatrics offers a more scaled-down estimate, claiming that breastfeeding accounts for savings of between four hundred to five hundred dollars a year. One group of breastfeeding advocates even suggests that a mother should breastfeed for three years, then take the three thousand dollars she would have spent over this time on formula and invest it in a trust fund at 8 or 9 percent long-term interest. By the time her child turns twenty-one, the initial three-thousand-dollar investment will have increased well into a five-figure number. The fact of the matter is simply this: Bottle-feeding costs a good deal of money. Breastfeeding is free.

Other general benefits of breastfeeding for mothers. Small benefits are benefits still. Here is a list of the little dividends and pleasing advantages that breastfeeding mothers gain.

- ౩ Breastfed babies smell better than bottle fed babies. Their skin seems softer to the touch, and more fragrant.
- ౩ The bowel movements of nursed infants are less offensive than those of formula-fed children. The stools of an infant on solids can be especially foul, while a child of the same age who suckles continues to produce movements that are relatively inoffensive.

⟡ Breastfed babies do not spit up as often as formula-fed babies. This means fewer spotted clothes for mother to deal with and less work in the laundry.

⟡ Breastfed infants force their exhausted mothers to relax and let go. It is nature's way of slowing mothers and helping them to recuperate from the effort of giving birth. Breastfeeding mothers are literally coerced by nature to go with the flow.

⟡ A breastfeeding mother who must travel does not need to pack cans of formula and feeding apparatus in her suitcase. Breastfeeding mothers travel light.

⟡ Besides requiring a breast pump for working mothers, breast-feeding usually needs no special equipment—and how easy it is with all the beautiful and comfortable cotton nursing bras on the market today. Further, any mother can choose to stay with a bra not specified for nursing as long as it is cotton and as long as she purchases a larger size for comfort.

⟡ As an infant's nutritional and physical needs change, a mother's body senses these changes and makes appropriate adjustments in her milk automatically. This means that the composition of breast milk is subtly modifying itself day to day and that at any given moment it provides a growing infant with exactly the balance of nutrients it requires.

⟡ Breastfeeding raises the level of "good" (HDL) cholesterol in a nursing mother's bloodstream, providing protection against heart attack and stroke.

⟡ A breastfeeding mother has no need to get up in the middle of the night to cook formula and to bang her head in the dark while she's at it. With baby sleeping nearby, the breast is always at the ready; no preparation time is needed. If a child is sleeping with the parents, a mother does not even have to get out of bed. I can add from my own experience that waking up at night for the conventional "night bottle" and anticipating taking my turn for bottle-feeding duties concerned me during our pregnancy because I have grave difficulty falling back to sleep once I am awakened in the middle of the night. Knowing instead that our son had only to roll over silently to a welcoming mother whose breast was always available and whose embrace was a motor reflex even in her sleep allowed me to sleep through the night after Kesem was born without having guilty feelings that I was not pulling my share or that I was letting my wife down.

ᶘ Milk production burns up two hundred to five hundred calories a day in nursing mothers. To give you an idea what this figure means in terms of physical exertion, it takes more than an hour of treadmill walking at four miles an hour to burn five hundred calories. The result is simple: breastfeeding mothers tend to lose pregnancy weight faster than bottle-feeding mothers—that is, breastfeeding mothers tend to return more quickly to prepregnancy maintenance weights.

ᶘ Breastfeeding helps diabetic mothers. Those who suffer from diabetes return to their optimal weight more quickly than non-breastfeeding mothers, thus preventing a worsening of their condition. Diabetic mothers also need less insulin and medication for their condition while they are nursing.

ᶘ Breastfeeding can be done wherever mother happens to be, without the need for fumbling for feeding equipment and searching for the extra bottle she may have forgotten to pack in her bag. I recall one icy December when my son was two years old. It was freezing in New York City, and the streets were blanketed with snow. My wife, my son, and I were in a Korean market, shopping for groceries. While pushing past the produce counter, we heard my son's small, throaty sound that we recognized as a primary hunger cue. My wife responded immediately: Without even slowing the shopping cart, she discretely and easily embraced our son, who was hanging in a sling close to her breast. Here, I thought, was yet another example of how breastfeeding allows us to go on with ease and dignity in the midst of everyday life.

⟫ The fact that nursing women do not have a monthly cycle provides them with a decreased risk of iron-deficiency anemia, which is so common in non-breastfeeding women. The longer a mother nurses and keeps her periods at bay, the stronger this effect becomes.

⟫ A breastfeeding mother has no need to fill her shelves with plastic bottles, metal formula cans, rubber nipples, and the like. This translates into a reduction in a town or city garbage dump of the PCBs and nonbiodegradable items that are part of bottle-feeding. Breastfeeding is good for the environment as well as for the people living in it.

The Importance of Bonding and Breastfeeding to the Family

All too often public health agencies advocate for breastfeeding on purely medical grounds: Breastfeeding reduces colds in a child. It provides natural immunities. It builds a well-formed palate and bite.

Yet while these claims are true, as we have seen, somewhere in their reports these agencies fail to spell out the intensely powerful emotional impact that breastfeeding produces in mother and child. Writes Dr. Alicia Dermer, "In Western society, the decision about breast or bottle is still seen very much as a personal choice based on convenience. The potential stress of living with a child with recurrent illnesses, or the loss of the unique bond that comes from breastfeeding, are often omitted from the decision-making process."[45]

The bond that Dr. Dermer refers to begins at the moment skin-to-skin contact is made between a nursing mother's body and the child's. It seems nothing could be more intimate than the nursing position itself: the child is pressed tightly against the mother's warm torso; its little mouth is latched onto an erect but pliable nipple as it sucks a warm, delicious substance that only enhances the child's sense of safety and well-being. We have only to imagine the smoothness of skin against skin; the aromas emitted by bodies; the presence of a loving father nearby, holding the nursing mother in a warm embrace as she brings food and nurturance to their child. Here is a united trio of lovers and beloved.

Throughout this book we have sung the praises of the remarkable partnership that can take shape between a mother and a child in utero, at birth, and beyond and which is referred to simply as *bonding*. Here, bonding occurs via the route of nursing. The fact of the matter is that of all the elements in the bonding process, none brings mother and child closer together than this act. When a baby is hungry, a nursing mother is there with the breast immediately, without the need to fumble with bottles and cooked formula.

Such instant gratification increases a child's mood and sense of control over the surrounding environment, which sends the message that the world is a good and safe place; the world will provide and nurture— don't worry. The insistence that children be fed according to a rigid hourly schedule day and night rather than on demand seems cold and hard in light of breastfeeding's affirmative benefits. Certainly, it appears to be of no help in bolstering a hungry newborn's trust of its parents, who appear to withhold food on an arbitrary basis and who deny a child the calming body comforts that come with skin-on-skin, mouth-to-nipple contact.

According to Dr. William Sears in his book *The Womanly Art of Breastfeeding:*

> Breastfeeding mothers respond to their babies more intuitively and with less restraint. The baby's signals of hunger or distress trigger a biological response within the mother (a milk let-down), and she feels the urge to pick up the baby and nurse her. This response rewards both mother and baby with good feelings. If a mother is bottle-feeding, her response to her baby crying is quite different. She must initially divert her attention away from the baby to an object,

the bottle, and take time to find and prepare it. As you recall, a baby's memory span in the first six months is from four to ten seconds. The time it takes to produce a nonbiological response, such as bottle-feeding, is usually longer than the baby's memory span. The bottle-feeding baby does not receive the same immediate reinforcement of his cues that a breastfeeding baby does. In my practice, I have noticed that breastfeeding mothers tend to show a high degree of sensitivity to their babies, and I believe this is a result of the biological changes that occur in a mother in response to the signals of her baby.[46]

As we have seen, on a somatic level the elements of touch, smell, and warm temperature trigger the flow of the hormone oxytocin in the mother's bloodstream. Via breastfeeding, this hormone then passes into the child. Here, oxytocin begins to weave a complex, magical spell on both parties, increasing the mother's sense of protection for her infant, reducing stress, speeding up the mother's healing, lowering blood pressure and adrenalin levels in her blood, generating a pleasant sedative effect in mother and child alike, and triggering thunderous bursts of love and affection between mother and child.

Meanwhile, while oxytocin performs its wonders, the other principal birth chemical, the "mothering hormone" prolactin, kicks in around the end of the first week after birth, after colostrum has done its job. Prolactin goes to work immediately manufacturing milk, and ensuring that this milk is perfectly balanced with the child's needs. On an emotional level, prolactin stimulates a mother's maternal instincts, relaxing her, promoting sound sleep, and causing her to bond more intimately with the newborn. The baby's continual sucking stimulates further prolactin release, which makes more milk, which is then sucked up again, which then generates still more milk—the entire process turns the breasts into a perpetual milk-making machine that can be shut down only if the mother or the infant should have health problems or until the infant weans. All this interior hormonal activity is the mechanism that drives the suckling impulse and gives it such an emotional power as well as a physiological boost.

An interesting point about prolactin: hormonal studies—which are often made in developing countries, where men often play a far larger role in caring for children than in modern industrial cultures—show that when a father is close to his infant or is near his partner who is nursing their child, his testosterone level drops (testosterone fosters aggressive behavior) and his prolactin levels increase dramatically. In one African tribe, for instance, prolactin levels were found to be five times higher than normal among men who carried their infant regularly and helped out with childcare.

BREASTFEEDING FOR WORKING MOTHERS

Breastfeeding can be relatively easy for stay-at-home mothers—but what about mothers who work? Must a working mother and her newborn be denied the benefits and pleasures of breastfeeding, including the bonding that breastfeeding brings?

The answer: not at all. Working mothers are not denied this right. For them, breastfeeding simply requires becoming educated in the ways of nursing a child while working out of the home.

For starters, the growing support of employers across the country, plus a variety of new and innovative milk storage aids, make breastfeeding on the job a more viable option than at any other time in history. Before a mother begins her maternity leave, she first must ask if there is a lactation policy offered at her place of work. Interested mothers should find out if their employers allow mothers to bring a newborn to work to breastfeed on the premises. Many employers now offer this and some even provide private quarters for these sessions. Women and men might even let employers know that they stand to benefit from mothers who breastfeed on the job; statistically, mothers who breastfeed miss work far less frequently than those who bottle feed.

If children are not allowed to stay with mothers all day at work, perhaps the childcare provider taking care of the infant at home can bring the child to the office several times a day for feeding. If this is not possible, the mother should be able to leave and go nurse the child. In such a scenario, the mother takes the child to a private place for ten or fifteen minutes, feeds her baby, then returns to work. An increasing number of companies now oblige new mothers in this regard.

Mothers-to-be can also inquire about the possibility of working at home several days a week or if working part-time for, say, six months, is a possibility. This would guarantee a child a respectable amount of time at the breast. If it is not possible for a mother to bring her child to work or to have a childcare provider bring the child to her, she should take full advantage of her maternity leave to establish a good supply of milk before returning to work. Remember: the longer you stay home and concentrate on breastfeeding your baby, the easier it will be to maintain your milk supply after you reenter the labor force.

A working mother's biggest foe, regardless of how she chooses to feed her infant: fatigue. One way to reduce it: Return to work the first week on a Thursday rather than on a Monday. Then take the next two Wednesdays as sick or personal leave days so that you are not working more than two days in a row. This schedule will get you back into the swing of work gradually, giving you and your baby more time to adjust to modifications in routine. On weekends or days off, breastfeed your baby as often as possible. Remember that it is normal for your milk supply to decline toward the end of a workweek. Breastfeeding as frequently as possible on weekends and relaxing in the process will help you to recharge and increase your milk surplus for the coming week.

Once a mother does return to work, she can nurse her baby immediately before leaving home, then express milk at work at the baby's usual feeding time and have this milk picked up by the caregiver in charge of the infant. A breast pump that is chosen carefully will enable a mother to collect and store milk at work for feedings she will miss at home. Automatic-cycling, hospital-type electric pumps provide a safe, fast, efficient way to express milk from the breasts. Note too that breast milk stays fresh in a refrigerator for forty-eight hours and if frozen, maintains its integrity for up to three months. Many mothers pump extra supplies of milk, freeze them, then use them as needed.

Another way of dealing with at-work breastfeeding: a childcare provider brings the infant to work at lunchtime, when a mother can feed it during this gap in the work day. In this scenario, the baby is breastfed in the morning and again at lunchtime. A childcare provider can then use pumped breast milk for an afternoon feeding. When a mother and baby are reunited in the evening, they can breastfeed to their heart's content.

DALIT'S EXPERIENCE

In the beginning, I was embarrassed by what I thought other women would think, and I was also conscious of the prying eyes of men, who in our culture do not regard the breast as a nurturing object, but rather as a sexual object. But as I stared back directly into the curious eyes of both men and women, the knowledge that was exchanged in a single glance let me know that on some deeper level, I was respected. This encouraged me and helped me quickly to get past my self-consciousness and embarrassment.

THE FATHER'S ROLE
AND NURSING THE WORLD

When mothers look back at their breastfeeding years, many consider them to be a very special time in their lives—but it is important to remember that the father plays his part in the process as well, encouraging and nurturing the mother in her natural child rearing ventures.

This is especially true if the father gives his unconditional support to the process of breastfeeding, doing all he can to help his wife in her endeavors to feed and otherwise help their child. Indeed, a picture of partners and child is this: The mother feeds the child and the father simultaneously feeds the mother in a perfectly balanced and unending rondo. All three then spread the joy of this harmonious union to other members of the family, to their friends and neighbors, and, by some indefinable way, to strangers they have not yet met—for joy, like its dark counterforces of despair, anger, and depression is infectious. Every man, woman, and child it touches is enriched and made glad.

⌒

It is critical to realize that though breastfeeding keeps mother, father, and child healthy, bonded, and affectionate, there is another unsung and difficult-to-measure benefit to society at large. Common sense tells us that men and women who have passed their infancy and childhood in vibrant mental and emotional health, bonded to both parents, and secure in the physical and emotional love of those around them will grow up to be well-adjusted, productive adults. A sound mind and sound body grow only if these patterns are set for children in their earliest days. This is how we help to create tolerant, creative, and kindly human beings.

Breastfeeding, then, is one more way in which parents can help to fix the world.

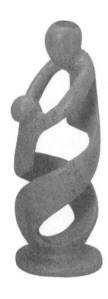

6

Life after Birth

The Most Important
Days of Our Lives

*In kin-based communities, women who adhere to
customary postpartum rituals seldom experience
postpartum depression. The need for postpartum rituals
is filled among Jewish families, if a son is born, by the
traditional bris, and among many Christian families by
the christening ceremony followed by a party.*

*But for the many who do not practice such religious
rituals, friends and/or family could provide effective rituals
of reintegration. There could be tremendous benefit for
new mothers if a postpartum baby-welcoming party were to
become as standard as the pre-birth baby shower.*

HARRIET ROSENBERG, "MOTHERWORK,
STRESS AND DEPRESSION," 1987

A WORD ABOUT
POSTPARTUM DEPRESSION

Postpartum depression is a very real thing. In our modern American society the new mother is often isolated during her maternity leave.

Even if she is a powerful executive in the workplace, she is now at home feeling overwhelmed and uninformed about how to cope with this wonderful, but challenging newborn. Her world has changed dramatically, and frankly women who suffer from postpartum depression are criticized and made to feel even worse about themselves. It can be a time of marital strife and family conflict. It is absolutely essential for the new mother to receive support from her partner, family, and friends. We urge new parents to contact a local parenting group or the LeLeche League in your area. Ask your pediatrician, midwife, or family physician for information. A new mother who is severely depressed feels guilty because she cannot feel the tremendous joy that everyone talks about. She fears that she is a bad mother if she has feelings of resentment. Happy parents make happy kids, so please seek help if you are feeling depressed. It is nothing to be ashamed of and it is not your fault. Everyone deserves to have a joyful experience during this precious time of your life. It is normal for a new mother to feel "a little blue" due to hormonal changes, but if you are feeling sad for more than a few days please reach out and get help!

DRINKING FROM THE RIVER LETHE

It is impossible for us to understand fully how a newborn child perceives and evaluates the universe around it. Like souls in the Greek underworld who drink from the River Lethe then forget all that happened to them on earth, so we as grown men and women experience a kind of amnesia: We forget everything we experienced during the first hours, days, and months of our infancy.

The irony behind this dreamy blackout is that our days and months of infancy are supremely critical in forming the attitudes we bring into adulthood and in structuring the very roots of our personality.

We can only imagine what it is like to be a newborn. We can picture them, just arrived in this world. Perhaps it is the second week after birth. They see enormous, smiling heads gazing down, some wearing bizarre expressions and laughing with a rumble that must sound like thunder to the newly born. An infant's senses perceive the bed it lies in is as a great expanse—as large as a huge room is to our perception. The light that shines from a nearby table lamp blazes as brightly as an incandescent star. Everything for newborns—neonates, as they are called in obstetric language—is new and alien: colors, sounds, and movements; the smell of milk and the mother's warm body; the taste of food; a sudden draft of summer air; the first tactile contact with wool, metal, and earth; the first bath. All of these are familiar objects and experiences that the habituated senses of adults take for granted, but to the newborn's elemental yet keen observations, all of these appear marvelous and fresh. For the first time, the second time, and even the third time, these sensory contacts with reality are wondrous to the child's perceptions—but we parents and adults must also remember that they can be overwhelming and at times menacing. Whatever form they take—positive, neutral, or negative—they leave messages that are imprinted as clearly on a newborn's nervous system as they might be carved in a piece of wood.

A unique and uncanny description of how infants perceive the brave new world they are entering is described in *Tales of Power,* by Carlos Castaneda. After attending graduate school at the department of ethnology at UCLA in the 1960s, Castaneda claimed to have apprenticed himself to a Yaqui Indian shaman in Mexico while working on his doctorate. He reported that he spent several years at his master's side studying ancient Indian sorcery and spirituality, then eventually wrote a series of bestselling books blending scientific anthropology and exotic adventure with a startling and, for some, credibility-stretching mysticism. Most people who have read one or more of these works, however—whether they consider them fact or simply imaginative storytelling—concede that they are full of unique insights and keen psychological observations. Particularly revealing in *Tales of Power* is one of Castaneda's autobiographical passages, which, he tells us, he recalled while in a state of expanded consciousness induced in him by his shaman teacher. Whether such an event actually occurred or is simply the author's imagination at play, we can sense an accuracy in his description that speaks to our own unconscious memories.

The sequence starts with Castaneda going into a kind of blackout, then waking up to find himself lying on an enormous floor composed of beautiful, symmetrical slabs of an unknown material. As he attempts to roll over and sit up, he discovers he has no control over his body. He is inert and has no sense of any of his anatomical parts being connected to the others. He can only sway, wobble, and move his head limply from side to side. When he looks down at his limbs, they appear distorted and foreign, as if he is studying the body of another person.

Gazing upward, he sees a large sun directly overhead in a yellow sky. It casts a warm, dull glow. He is able to stare into it without discomfort. A moment later he finds himself being shaken violently, then picked up by a giant, barefoot female and carried across the room as if he is a doll. Hanging limply over her shoulder and looking down at the floor as they walk, he sees the girl's feet making huge pressure marks on the patterned slabs that give elastically under her tremendous weight.

The giant female places him on his stomach in front of a huge buildinglike structure that he cannot identify. The structure has four columns that seem to hold up nothing in particular; they are long and perfectly proportioned obelisks that tower upward toward the yellow sky. The effect of this beautiful sight causes him to enter a state of rapture.

Then suddenly another woman enters the room. She is much larger than the first—so immense that her body eclipses the light from the sun overhead. The gigantic female seems angry. She takes hold of the columned structure and turns it upside down. It is a chair! Castaneda writes: "The realization was like a catalyst. It triggered some overwhelming perceptions. . . . I realized that the magnificent and incomprehensible floor was a straw mat; the yellow sky was the ceiling of a room; the sun was a light bulb. The structure that had evoked such rapture in me was a chair that the child had turned upside down to play house."[1]

The child, it turns out, is Castaneda's older sister, who played with him when they were both very young. The giant woman was his mother.

THE POWER OF PARENTAL NURTURANCE

The episode that Castaneda describes is perhaps akin to experiences that we also underwent as infants at a time when our unconditioned minds scanned the world with no preconceptions and no data bank of past experience to help us identify even the most familiar objects around us.

Whatever children see at this stage of development passes directly into parts of their highly suggestible mammalian brain, which in early infancy remains uninfluenced by the yet-unformed ego. The child does not attempt to make familiar that which is unfamiliar. It has no expectations of how the world should be or look or behave. Instead, the newborn simply accepts what it sees as what is, avoiding all attempts, as Joseph Chilton Pearce phrases it, "to squeeze experience into a tight frame of stable reference."[2]

The fact is that the two angels with fiery swords who guard the gateway of our unconscious have not yet taken their places in our minds at this early stage—that is, we have not yet formed the ego desires, defense mechanisms, and Pavlovian responses we use as adults to exclude unpleasant information and classify the world into tidy categories. Our psychological firewalls and secret rooms and fortifications remain unconstructed. As a matter of course, then, we remain wide open psychologically and emotionally, allowing these initial impressions to emblazon themselves on the deepest layers of our unconscious minds, where they serve as the ground-floor building blocks in the rising citadel of our developing consciousness.

For this reason and for many others, the events that usher us into the first minutes, hours, days, and weeks after birth are in many ways the most important days of our lives. We know this through studies of newborns and by studies of how immediate post-birth experiences affect children and how these children fare in the months and years that follow birth. The theme that runs through these studies is that the many nurturing activities that parents perform for their children—some of which will be presented in this chapter—fall under a single umbrella concept that we have seen before: bonding.

Throughout this book we have seen how bonding begins in utero and how it influences children at the moment of birth and throughout breastfeeding. In this chapter we explore other ways that bonding can be nurtured in a newborn's life as it works to assimilate all that surrounds it.

Based on the most compelling obstetric and psychological evidence currently available, included in this chapter is information that parents can adopt to ensure that their newborn child receives crucial advantages, which so many infants in our day are denied. What can be done at the key moments after birth are quite practical: the small effects we produce with our hands, eyes, voice, body, and environment—those ways of interacting that bring an observable positive response—can determine a child's destiny.

Some of these suggestions and methods are obvious, and some are not. Some are easy to apply, while others take work or at least time, plus a willingness to run counter to popular wisdom that has often interfered with the fundamental biological imperatives that are so necessary for a child's sound development. None of these methods are new; they are as old as time—simple, traditional, and often self-evident nurturing techniques that, for one reason or another, have been swept away from the modern nursery and made obsolete by a system pressured by the stresses of modern living.

THE SCIENTIFICATION OF LOVE

In the short, information-rich overview of bonding entitled *The Scientification of Love,* French medical writer and researcher Michel

Odent provides an encapsulated explanation of how the circuit of love that flows between mother and newborn (and on a larger scale, between romantic lovers and even close friends) operates behind the scenes—more or less "in the boiler room," on a hormonal and unconscious level.

According to Odent, parental bonding is simply love in action, while love is potentially parental bonding: the two, he tells us, are one and the same but viewed from different perspectives. He also tells us why and how this magical welding of hearts—this bonding—must take place right away in a child's life, in the hour of birth and in the days and weeks that follow. If these bonding activities are absent, Odent warns, there is disruption in the genetic scenario that eons of evolution have engineered into infants for their harmonious growth and development.

We know that a child learns basically from what it sees and experiences, not from what it is told. It requires a visible model to jump-start the hormonal aids that nature has built into the hard wiring of its being. A salmon, studies confirm, is hormonally hard-wired to swim upstream and mate, but it will do so only if it sees other salmon performing the same journey. The early mother-child bonding exchange is similar. The care and nurturance—or lack of these—that newborns see and feel from their parents become a primary determinant not only of how well these children mature, but also of how successfully they will one day parent and love their own offspring.

Odent writes:

> Of all the different manifestations of love—maternal, paternal, filial, sexual, romantic, platonic, spiritual, brotherly love, not to mention love of country, love of inanimate objects, and compassion and concern for mother earth—the prototype of all these ways of loving is *maternal love*. What is more, the evidence points to a short and yet critical period of time just after birth, which has long-term consequences so far as our future capacity to love is concerned. We disregard the consequences of ritualizing, interfering with, or otherwise neglecting the physiology of that critical period at our peril.[3]

In chapter 3, we discussed the place that body chemistry plays in childbirth and how the "hormonal cocktail," shaken and stirred during the hours of birth and before, plays so many simultaneous roles in helping nature's birth plan unfold with a minimum of danger and discomfort. Scientific awareness of how this plan works began in 1968, when Terkel and Rosenblatt segregated a group of virgin female rats and injected them with the blood of mother rats that had given birth within the past forty-eight hours. The experimenters noted that the injected rats immediately began to exhibit maternal behavior toward baby mice that were not their own. Maternal love, it seems, can be traced to a chemical—several chemicals, in fact—that reside in the blood.[4]

It is also clear, Odent tells us, that the different hormones released by mother and baby during labor and delivery are not eliminated from their systems immediately. After birth they tend to linger, continuing to exert important affects on the maternal relationship.

As we have discovered, oxytocin, the so-called hormone of love, stimulates uterine contractions during birth and helps parents work together lovingly during delivery. Yet its presence in the mother's body immediately following birth is also critical. Among other post-delivery functions, the love hormone triggers the emotions of tenderness and attachment between mother and child that are so decisive in early attachment parenting. Prolactin, another birth hormone that lingers in the mother's body, regulates breastfeeding and appears to exert a positive effect on the newborn's developing immune system. When breastfeeding takes place, prolactin acts as a natural contraceptive, suppressing the ovulatory cycle at a time when pregnancy would be a disastrous event for all involved. As we have seen, we know that breastfeeding is 90 percent effective as a contraceptive during the first month of a child's life. We also know that during the birth process, mother and child produce morphine-like hormones that remain in their systems for a time after birth, raising the endorphin levels so important for happiness and relief of pain, but also supporting the act of mutual attunement between mother and child. "The property of opiates to induce states of dependency is well known," writes Odent. "So it is easy to anticipate how the beginning of a 'dependency'—an attachment—will be likely to begin."[5]

Finally, the adrenalin rush that takes place during birth, giving the mother extra energy and alertness to deliver her child, remains in the body of the child. Here, it serves the purpose of keeping the child alert with eyes wide open, allowing both parties to make prolonged and intense eye contact that, as we shall see, is a critical element in stimulating a loving bond between mother and child.

LACK OF BONDING: THE ROOTS OF DISEASE, ALIENATION, AND HUMAN VIOLENCE

As we know, modern obstetric procedures—the epidural, machine monitoring, the c-section, the use of tranquilizers—often suppress the natural deployment of these important birth hormones, sometimes to a significant degree. When these obstetric procedures are used, results can have a significant impact on the newborn and the child it grows to become. In several fascinating chapters and referring to a wide number of controlled studies, Odent spells out the negative consequences in dismaying sequence.

✤ **Youthful violence.** A team of doctors at the University of California in Los Angeles studied 4,269 males born in a Denmark hospital. Tracking the history of these males over the years, they found that the main risk factor for youthful crime stemmed from birth complications—but only if coupled with rejection by the mother at birth or by the early separation of mother and child.[6]

✤ **Autism.** Autistic children have no ability to bond with other human beings or interact socially either with children or adults. They are incapable of making meaningful eye contact and often cannot speak at all. Many seriously autistic people spend their lives watching endless hours of TV or performing ritual behaviors.

In one study a Japanese researcher found that the incidence of autism among children born in a certain hospital was abnormally high. It also turned out that this hospital induced labor routinely in mothers who were a week before their due date and that during labor, it regularly used an assortment of obstetric procedures and medications, including sedatives, anesthesia, and analgesics.[7]

Researchers Niko and Elizabeth Tinbergen studied autistic children for many years, concluding that specific obstetric procedures contribute to this condition. These include deep forceps delivery, anesthesia at birth, resuscitation at birth, the artificial induction of labor, and the lack of eye contact between mother and child that results when newborns are separated from their mothers immediately after delivery.[8]

A number of other studies around the world have reached similar conclusions. Writes Odent:

> The results of the main studies which have detected links between how people are born and different forms of impaired capacity to love have been published in very authoritative medical journals. However, they are comparatively unknown and are not taken into account in most subsequent articles. One might also wonder why most of these studies were not repeated by a greater number of researchers.[9]

✦ **Teenage suicide.** Teenage suicide in the United States was literally unknown before World War II. Today, it is epidemic. Odent cites studies establishing a relationship between methods used by teenagers to kill themselves and early birth traumas. Studies show that in a large number of cases, suicide by asphyxiation is linked to a child's inability to breath during the first few moments after birth. Suicide using mechanical means is associated with mechanical birth trauma due to interventions with obstetric equipment. Horrendously violent methods of self-destruction are associated closely with the fact that the mothers of suicide victims used opiate painkillers while in labor and immediately after. A large number of drug-addicted teenagers show a similar correlation.

✤ **Unwanted child syndrome.** A team of researchers in Gothenburg, Sweden, studied the lives of children whose mothers had been unsuccessful in their applications to the state for abortions. Researchers monitored the 120 subjects plus a control group of the same number to the age of twenty-one. The main conclusion was that in adulthood the unwanted children were far less capable of socializing and forming lasting relationships than those in the control group. Like studies have come to similar conclusions.[10]

Many other studies suggest strongly that medical interventions at birth and immediately thereafter can and often do cause long term deficits in children. To counteract this, parents can use many practical techniques recommended by enlightened childcare professionals around the world who know the value of new parenting methods. This help begins the moment newborns are out of the womb. For information on the best time to cut the umbilical cord as well as on what may happen if the cord is cut too soon, see chapter 4.

THE FIVE FUNDAMENTAL NEEDS OF A CHILD IMMEDIATELY FOLLOWING BIRTH

According to Joseph Chilton Pearce in *Magical Child Matures,* in order for the bonding process to proceed seamlessly, five basic sensory-motor functions must be awakened and set to work in a child immediately following birth. Each of these functions corresponds to one of the five senses. Writes Pearce:

> The job of birthing is to activate this sensory system in its entirety, and get the processing of information functional in the shortest possible time. . . . The infant cannot provide himself with any of this sensory activation after delivery. All of it must be done *for* the newborn, and his system is designed with the expectation that this will *be* done. . . . The inner blueprints of sight, sound, touch, taste, and

smell will then be given their necessary stimulus, their model content, from the physical world, anchoring the bonding bridge in the new domain. The necessary functional structure of brain/mind and body will rapidly unfold, and birth will be complete.[11]

While each of these functions is switched on in a different way, Pearce tells us, all five require a single, universal action to trigger them: placing the newborn infant in physical contact with the mother. Pearce goes on to say: "Activation of the senses takes place automatically and spontaneously simply by introducing the infant to the mother in skin-to-skin contact immediately after delivery. Millions of years of biological encoding ensure the instinctive response of each to the other from this point on."[12]

Once enclosed in this maternal cornucopia of warmth and affection, the infant's brain starts to receive signals that the trillion-celled kingdom over which it is destined to rule is waking up—time to get to work! Once the sensory reflexes of the neonate are activated, the brain starts relaying its own neurological messages, and infant development moves out of first gear into second and third. Life accelerates.

In his famous work *Man on His Nature*, Charles Sherrington describes the brain activity of a person waking from sleep. His passage could as easily be used to describe the first waking of the neonate brain:

The great topmost sheet of the brain, that where hardly a light had twinkled or moved, becomes now a sparkling field of rhythmic flashing points with trains of traveling sparks hurrying hither and thither. The brain is starting to work, and with it the mind is returning. It is as if the Milky Way entered upon some cosmic dance. Swiftly the head becomes an enchanted loom where millions of flashing shuttles weave a dissolving, yet meaningful pattern, though never an abiding one; a shifting harmony of sub-patterns. Now as the waking body rises, sub-patterns of this great harmony of activity stretch down into the unlit tracts of the brain stalk. This means that the body is up and rises to meet its waking day.[13]

Now, while this post-birth sensory dance is taking place, the adrenal glands continue dutifully to pump adrenalin into the child's bloodstream in order to keep the infant aware and awake long enough to make eye contact with the mother and begin breastfeeding. As they pump, the adrenals wait patiently for an order from the brain to shut down. Once these glands are quieted, the newborn can then settle into a gentle sleep, its sensory functions operative and the first all-important few minutes of bonding with the mother completed.

If a newborn is whisked off to the nursery immediately after birth, however, and is prevented from making prolonged skin-to-skin contact with the mother, nature's built-in neurological plan becomes sabotaged. None of the chemical reactions that are programmed into the child and that are timed to go off as soon as mother-child physical contact is made are not activated. Consequently, a shutdown message is never sent to the adrenals and the brain fails to deliver instructions to the baby's five senses concerning what to do next. Without this cease-and-desist order from the chief, adrenalin continues to pool in the child's system until it reaches a critical mass. Eventually, it sends the infant into various degrees of shock. Statistically, if the five sensory faculties are not aroused via contact with the mother within approximately forty-five minutes after delivery and if the adrenalin flow is not quelled during this time, the infant's sensory-motor system closes down, reverting to a prebirth, uterine state of consciousness. If this occurs, infants really do become the insensate, somnambulistic blobs that earlier developmental psychologists thought they were. The infant's natural adaptation to the world, which should be galloping ahead, instead comes to a halt—or perhaps we should say that it never gets out of the starting gate.

Conversely, what happens physically and psychologically when infant and mother make their first body-to-body and heart-to-heart contact following birth? How are the five sensory reflexes—so critical to the development of the child's intelligence, physical prowess, and mental health—stimulated and aroused?

Let us take a close look at how, when mother and child are allowed to make contact, each of these five sensory-motor reflexes are set in motion and primed to operate for the next eighty or ninety years.

The Sense of Sight

For centuries it has been assumed that infants are born blind. I remember being solemnly informed of this fact by my father when my own baby brother was born. "Don't try to make him laugh like that, Jeffrey," my father warned. "He can't see you. He probably can't hear you either." Friends of my own generation remember similar dictums from their parents.

The truth is that not only can newborns see, but also that they see in a special way that ensures that they survive and increases their ability to bond. Newborn eyes are engineered by nature's post-birth program to focus on whatever is in front of them from a distance of eight to twelve inches. This distance, significantly, is the approximate space that separates the mother's face and that of the child when the child lies on the mother's chest. It is also the approximate distance between the child's mouth and the mother's nipple in the nursing position.

Once placed on the mother's chest in the moments following birth, infants start to look for the nipple automatically. When they see it with their eight-to-twelve-inch gaze, aided by their sense of smell, they crawl toward it, and feeding soon begins. Assuming that the newborn's other body functions are working properly, its chances of survival are now made certain. This is the practical and biological function of newborn sight. On an emotional level, an even more profound type of seeing takes place that helps a newborn function at its full feeling potential.

We know that among adults, staring into another person's eyes for prolonged periods is tricky business. Intense staring occurs normally if two people are romantically attracted or, ironically, if they are about to come to blows. The saying "he blinked first" means that the other person broke eye contact and thus backed down from an intimate—or combative—confrontation. According to optometric studies, eye contact between strangers lasting longer than a second and a half is considered invasive and inappropriate—or is simply an invitation to flirt.

Interestingly, the gaze that takes place between mother and child immediately after birth is much like the exchange of amorous glances that passes between lovers. Recall Michel Odent's profound statement that maternal love is the prototype of all ways of loving. At the same time, the locked eyes of mother and child serve as a biological pump that accelerates secretions of the love hormone oxytocin into the bloodstream of each of the two parties. Mutual gazing likewise stimulates other hormones that play a role in cementing maternal attachment.

Because these hormones escalate a mother's adoration for her newborn to transcendent levels, kindling feelings of loyalty, nurturance, and protection in the process, mutual gazing is nature's way of bestowing a triple blessing:

1. The newborn's ability to organize visual data is activated.
2. The mother undergoes states of rapture and communion.
3. The mother's protective and nurturing instincts are raised to maximum levels. In the process, the survival rate among newborn human beings, and hence of the human race, is increased dramatically.

Studies show that mutual gazing likewise increases heartbeat, breathing rate, and galvanic skin response. When tested, mothers and children who make prolonged early eye contact also show an unusually high level of happiness-inducing endorphins in their bloodstreams. Studies suggest that fathers who make intense eye contact with newborns also increase their chances of enjoying a warm, intimate relationship with their child. Indeed, some research suggests that eye-gazing infants grow up especially close to their parents and remain connected with them in a positive, healthy way.

There is, however, a caveat connected to the visual response mechanism of newborns—or rather, to the lack of this mechanism. Writes Gwyneth Doherty-Sneddon in her book *Children's Unspoken Language:*

> One study found that babies who did not make mutual eye contact with their caregivers in their first month of life had rather difficult patterns of subsequent development compared with those who did. For example, early "nongazers" generally showed developmental delay, and had more behavioral problems at age six years than those who did engage in early mutual gaze.[14]

To these observations, Joseph Chilton Pearce adds the equally tragic fact that a drugged mother and a drugged baby will be incapable of using their eyes for any type of mutual gazing, thereby losing this precious opportunity for early bonding. Indeed, the brains of children born under heavy sedation may temporarily lose their ability to organize visual stimuli into recognizable faces of any kind. This ability, Pearce warns, often does not return to the child for several months after birth.[15]

Keeping all this in mind, new parents are encouraged to make eye contact with their newborn as frequently as possible, and to do so from the moment the child is born through the first year of infancy. For a mother, breastfeeding is an especially appropriate time for contented gazing. For a father, cradling a newborn in his arms and smiling down on it is all that is required. The important thing is simply to do it.

The Sense of Hearing

Almost the moment that infants are born and placed on their mother's chests, they begin to crawl slowly but inexorably toward the mother's left breast. Because newborns are entirely immobile for the first few weeks of life and appear to have no coordination between their hands and feet, the fact that they actually crawl this distance is a mysterious miracle unto itself. Whatever the explanation, the crawling reflex exists clearly to help the child reach the breast and commence feeding. Concurrently, though, something else is transpiring in this mini drama.

We can note that the child almost always crawls instinctively to the left breast, never to the right. Interestingly, the left breast is located over the heart. With its ear planted next to its mother's chest, a nursing infant can hear the resonant sound of the heart's beating—the same sound they listened to day and night in the womb for nine straight months. Blood tests in infants show that the sound of this rhythm raises endorphin levels and strengthens immunity. The synchronization of the mother's heartbeat and the child's breathing patterns, moreover, stimulates and balances developing metabolism. Finally, on an emotional level, the closeness of the child to this sacred organ of life and love and the familiar pulsations it makes conjure up blissful feelings of peace and security, pulling ever tighter the strings that bind mother and child.

Another basic stimulus to the ear is the mother's voice. Even in the first moments following birth, an infant appears to respond to the love murmurings of parents. Tests show that newborns are able to identify their mother's voice quickly from among dozens of other voices in their surroundings. Talking to a newborn constantly is thus one of the most effective ways to activate its auditory senses and to increase the degree of communication and attachment between infant and parents. Though it may not seem as if infants are listening, in fact they are taking in every peep and syllable, processing it, and soon—perhaps sooner than you think—they begin to make sounds in return. With uncanny accuracy, some of these sounds mimic a mother's own sounds.

At the same time, the child's first sounds, the delightful blubbering and purring noises, trigger positive biological and psychological changes in the mother automatically. An increased quantity of blood flows to the breasts to stimulate breastfeeding and the mother's emotions are activated instantly, allowing feelings of love and attachment to pour forth. Intense moments of bonding follow on their own.

The Sense of Touch

The moment an infant emerges from the watery climate of the womb and makes contact with the warm flesh of the mother's body, the sensory reflex of touch is aroused. Billions of skin cells, nerves, and proprioceptors suddenly switch on, animating the child in a way that is analogous to God's touch of Adam in Michelangelo's famous Sistine Chapel panel.

Arguably, the sense of touch is the most primordial and pervasive of all physical sensations, and a newborn infant craves it almost as much as it craves food. The sense of touch grounds it to the new world around and to the people who love the newborn. From atop the mother's stomach immediately after birth, the newborn receives simultaneously everything it needs: warmth, protection, the breast, the sound of the mother's beating heart, and an intangible interchange of energies through the pores that create a sense of peace and security in both mother and child.

Because of this, it is vitally important that newborns not be separated from their mothers at birth. Not only should the two remain together during the first hours after birth, but they should be inseparable the entire length of time they are in the hospital. Dr. William Sears and hundreds of other doctors friendly to the new parenting thus advise that mother and child "room in"—that is, remain with each other during their entire hospital stay, making continual skin-on-skin connections. According to Dr. Sears, the following benefits are reaped from such togetherness:

❖ In the presence of the mother and by dint of the fact that a newborn is interacting with a single primary caregiver, it spends its first days feeling more content and secure.

❖ Rooming-in alters the priorities of attending hospital personnel, who, as a result, concentrate more fully on the care of the mother. The mother, in turn, is free to concentrate her care and affections entirely on the baby.

✤ The warm maternal touch plus the accompanying sense of the mother's smell, voice, and breast milk are known to reduce crying in newborns substantially and to synchronize the infant's sleep-waking cycle with that of the mother, producing better slumber for both.

✤ Breastfeeding runs more smoothly when mother and child are both in the same room. By constantly separating infants, then returning them to the mother, then taking them away again, a mother's flow of milk is slowed and a child's sucking reflex is dampened.

✤ It is not just the infant who suffers from separation anxiety. Mother's undergo their own form of this condition: They often feel restless and guilty. Rooming-in mothers, on the other hand, tend to be more relaxed, better rested, and less stressed. It is a myth, Sears insists, that the mothers of nursery-reared babies get better-quality rest. Studies show that quite the opposite is true.

✤ Rooming-in mothers experience a lower incidence of postpartum depression, and newborns have a considerably lower chance of developing jaundice.[16]

Skin temperature also plays a part in the magic domain of touch. Recent studies show that a child's inner body heat is warmer and better adjusted when it lies on the mother's body. Temperature charts indicate that if a newborn is taken away from its mother for more than a few minutes, its skin temperature begins to vacillate, rising one moment and falling the next. The skin temperature on a mother's chest, meanwhile, provides the baby with an extra degree of warmth than when the child is wrapped in a blanket. If the baby's temperature drops, the mother's skin temperature goes up one or two degrees to compensate. If the baby's skin surface is too warm, the mother's skin temperature drops a degree, cooling the newborn, a process known as *thermal synchrony.* Infant heart rate and breathing also improve on skin-to-skin contact. The heart beat becomes higher and more stable, the breathing is even and regular.[17]

Still another way in which skin contact activates a baby's sense of touch is by massage. Gently stroking and kneading a newborn's limbs, rubbing its stomach, and caressing its back and buttocks tend to wake the baby's senses, and at the same time such touch strengthens the bonds between mother and child. Massage also provides several essential mother-child bonding features: eye contact, skin-on-skin touch, proximity to the mother's smell, verbal exchanges, and so forth. Infant massage produces therapeutic benefits, increasing a newborn's lymph and blood flow, bringing relief from colic (and perhaps even preventing it), reducing stress and stimulating the digestive system and lowering the incidence of constipation and cramps. Nurturing touch also helps increase a child's weight gain and produces states of deep relaxation, promoting deeper and more satisfying sleep. Infant massage is an easy and joyous practice that induces pleasure in mother and child alike.

The Senses of Smell and Taste

When a newborn is first placed on its mother's chest, its sense of smell helps guide it to the nipple, where it begins to suckle. While some mothers help this process along by placing infants directly on the breast, even without this aid, if left to their own devices, neonates will follow the scented trail of milk and warmth directly to the mother's nipple. In most cases, no urging is required. Maternal smell and infant vision do all the work.

In laboratory tests, an infant demonstrates consistently the ability to recognize its mother's smell among the smell of other mothers. This is especially true if the infant is nursing. Moreover, an infant responds with positive behavior to its mother's odor, nursing more easily when detecting it and looking around the room with a gaze of contentment. Generally speaking, it takes about forty-five minutes for a baby to imprint on its mother's smell. If mother and child are separated during this time, a crucial bonding tool is lost.

Regarding taste, there are substances in mother's milk that stimulate growth hormones and activate taste reflexes in a newborn. It is believed that mother's milk also neutralizes excess amounts of adrenalin in the infant's systems, calming it and helping to bring its hormones into balance. "Frequent nursing," writes Pearce, "automatically ensures a major sensory stimulus on all levels: a constant renewal of the face at a distance of six to twelve inches, a renewal of the heartbeat connections; the familiar voice; and stimulus of the sensory endings of the skin by the continual movement of the mother in her daily routines."[18]

POST-BIRTH CLOSENESS

For many years, Western hospital protocol has demanded that newborns be taken away from their mothers and run through a gauntlet of medical procedures. By the time the mother is "allowed" to hold her baby, the precious forty-five-minute window of opportunity had often passed.

Today, happily, things have changed, and in many hospitals newborns are given over to the mother immediately following delivery. Even if a mother chooses not to deliver a newborn according to the principles of the new conscious parenting, the opportunity for post-birth closeness and bonding still exists. In it, a mother can perform the post-birth techniques described above, and further, parents can work with a hospital that allows rooming-in. The benefits of these simple acts can have profoundly positive effects on a newborn for the rest of its life.

THE PLEASURES AND
TREASURES OF CO-SLEEPING

In our age of euphemisms, the pleasant term "nighttime parenting," coined by Dr. William Sears, actually comes with several disguised recommendations. The most controversial of these, often heard from natural childcare advocates and pediatricians friendly to the new parenting techniques, is the suggestion that for the first few months following birth (and some would say for the first few years), it is best for children to co-sleep with their parents.

Around the turn of the century, Freud insisted that children who witness "the primal moment" accidentally—that is, those who catch sight of their parents making love—can become traumatized permanently, leading to a life of deep sexual confusion. As a result of this and other concerns, in our culture, the marriage bed is considered inviolate and anything that comes between spouses under the sheets is marked for removal. This "anything," of course, includes a child.

Also related to this taboo is the American axiom that children must become autonomous of their parents as quickly as possible. One month old is not too soon to begin. Independence is what this country was founded on, after all, and it is best for the new citizen to start off early. Moreover, regardless of how much the infant may kick, scream, and cry when placed in a separate room, parents are obliged to bite the bullet and maintain nighttime separation. Otherwise, as some experts insist, the child becomes spoiled, manipulative, and clingy. Insistent and, some might say, harsh means must therefore be applied when children attempt to insinuate themselves into the parental bed. "The parents have to be firm and committed to returning the child to bed," insists R. Ferber in his book *Solve Your Child's Sleep Problems.* "Parents have to learn to ignore crying until the child falls asleep. Sometimes children can cry for a couple of hours. Children may vomit with crying and so parents need to be prepared to go in and clean up the child and change the bedclothes quickly and, with the minimum of fuss, put the child back to bed, and walk out."[19]

Due to these and other cultural beliefs, the notion of an infant sleeping in the same bed with his or her mother and father is stigmatized with overtones of the sexual, the incestuous, and the overly dependent. Notwithstanding the fact that in most of the non-Western world, children sleep regularly in the same room or the same bed with their parents, apparently without suffering the traumatizing of witnessing "primal moments" (we will soon talk about the issue of co-sleeping and sexual privacy). Euro-American culture is decidedly opposed to such behavior, and in some cases, it is appalled at its mention. Yet in many countries, co-sleeping is considered mandatory for the health of the child, and the lack of it is looked on as a somewhat brutal error in basic parenting. Indeed, among the Japanese, where group harmony is considered an all-important goal, co-sleeping is part of the fabric of society. Caudil and Weinstein state:

> In Japan, the infant is seen more as a separate biological organism who from the beginning, in order to develop, needs to be drawn into increasingly interdependent relations with others. In America, the infant is seen as a dependent biological organism who in order to develop, needs to be made increasingly independent of others.[20]

Renowned psychologist T. Barry Brazleton adds, ". . . the Japanese think the U.S. culture rather merciless in pushing small children toward such independence at night."[21] According to an article in *Developmental Psychology,* women in southern Mexico and Guatemala, when informed that American babies are forced to sleep alone, responded with "shock, disapproval, and pity," thinking that this method is "tantamount to child neglect."[22]

We must note here that co-sleeping is not necessarily a make-it or break-it part of a child's formative life. Infants who sleep in a separate room, and who are otherwise bonded with their parents and well cared for in the new parenting style, tend to develop in normal, healthy ways. At the same time, studies show that co-sleeping may very well be an aid—perhaps a major one—for eliminating anxiety in newborns, accelerating the bonding process between parent and child, making nighttime breastfeeding more practicable, and giving the infant a sense of peacefulness and security.

According to pediatric research, then, what practical advantages result for parent and child from co-sleeping? Though the question is complex, it is worth noting the following experiments and observations, many of them performed at the Mother-Baby Behavioral Sleep Laboratory at the University of Notre Dame and from studies carried out there by James J. McKenna, Ph.D.

Greater sense of bonding, happiness, and safety. Imagine how much you as a three-year-old child would have preferred sleeping between your mother and father in one large bed rather than lying frightened and lonely in the exile of a separate room. No doubt, like most young children, you spent many long, dark nights crying for your parents.

Was this reaction an example of how "spoiled" you were at this age or how the development of your all-important independence would have been threatened if your parents "gave in" and allowed you to sleep in their room? Or did it simply reflect how profoundly you needed your mother and your father at this age during the precious hours of sleep— how much you needed their presence comforting you, warming you, loving you?

One cross-study of English children demonstrated that on a test scale, those prohibited from sleeping with their parents were more fearful than those who slept with at least one parent each night. The same researcher determined that solitary-sleeping children presented greater discipline problems when grown and dealt less proficiently with stress than those who were co-sleeping as children.[23]

A study of eighty-six children conducted on an army base showed that those who co-slept with their parents received better student evaluations from teachers than solitary-sleeping children. The authors of this study recorded that, "[c]ontrary to expectations, those children who had not had previous professional attention for emotional or behavioral problems co-slept more frequently than did children who were known to have had psychiatric intervention, and lower parental ratings of adaptive functioning."[24]

One of the largest studies on infant co-sleeping, carried out in New York and Chicago and involving more than fourteen hundred subjects taken from a rainbow of ethnic groups including Puerto Ricans, African-Americans, Dominicans, and Mexicans, found, among many positive results, that adults who were raised as infants sleeping in the same bed or room with their parents boasted extraordinarily strong feelings of happiness and satisfaction with life.[25]

Prevention of SIDS. For centuries, the terror of discovering their child dead in the crib for no apparent reason has haunted the dreams of parents. Today, studies show that SIDS is increasing in our society, and medical theories are constantly advanced to explain its mechanism.

According to recent studies, however, SIDS appears to be largely explainable, and in an extraordinarily simple way. "In fact," writes James McKenna, citing the work of Guntheroth and Spiers,[26] *"the sleeping position* of the infant has proven to be the single most important factor for reducing the chances of an infant dying of SIDS. . . . The discovery that merely placing infants in the supine [on the back] position, rather than in the prone [on the stomach] position, SIDS rates could decline as much as 90 percent in some countries continues to astonish many SIDS researchers worldwide."[27]

The fact is that while asleep, many infants migrate naturally to the prone position, but for biological and anatomical reasons this posture interferes with breathing and increases the chances of a stopping of breath. A parent who is present with a child throughout the night and who is aware subliminally of the infant's breathing patterns (studies show that most mothers instinctively awaken when their child stops breathing) and who periodically checks that the infant is sleeping in the supine position is also a parent who is actively guarding his or her child against the cessation of breathing that results in SIDS.

Other easily applied natural methods likewise appear to lower the incidence of SIDS. Writes McKenna:

> There are other parent-controlled "social" precautions that lower the risks of SIDS. Mitchell found that the presence of a responsible adult sleeping in the same room as an infant reduced by fourfold the chances of infants dying from SIDS. . . . Moreover, the largest epidemiological study to date conducted in Great Britain also shows increased risks for infants sleeping in rooms alone, as well as for babies sleeping in their mother's bed if the mother smokes. Other dangerous conditions include the use of duvets pulled over the

infant's head, and the use of soft mattresses. Overheating by over-wrapping an infant significantly increases SIDS risks. All this new data illustrate the extent to which infant sleep physiology is directly mediated by parental intervention.[28]

Other benefits of co-sleeping

Children who co-sleep cry less often than solitary sleepers.[29] Newborns who bed with their mothers also tend to breathe more deeply and suffer fewer periods of breath stoppage (known as obstructive apneas) that leads to respiratory complications and to SIDS. Additionally, as mentioned in chapter 4, while a mother is breastfeeding, having the infant close by at night makes it unnecessary to stumble out of bed from a deep sleep, stagger into another room, pick up the infant, and nurse while sitting in a chair or sofa. (Statistically, infants are most often dropped and injured at night by half-awake parents.) The co-sleeping child, lying comfortably in bed with the mother's nipple inches away, nurses more frequently and receives better nurturance and nourishment in the bargain.

We know that older children who share their parent's room wet their beds less often than children who sleep alone. Further, co-sleepers look with indifference on attachment objects such as blankets, stuffed animals, and dolls, which children adopt as surrogate guardians in the absence of a parent. The same is true for thumb sucking: the incidence of this disturbing habit is remarkably lower among co-sleepers than among children who slumber in a separate room. In one Turkish study of thumb sucking, 96 percent of children who sleep alone were found to suck their thumbs, while not a single infant practiced this habit in the control group of co-sleepers.[30]

According to one study, parents who are absent from home during the day find that co-sleeping allows them to compensate for their absence. One women interviewed in California remarked that "sleeping with my baby lets me make up some time I couldn't spend with her during the day, since my husband and I do not return to the house until early evening. Co-sleeping gives me more time to feel and nurture my baby."[31]

Co-sleeping and Parental Sex

An important question arises when we consider co-sleeping: What about making love when a child is sharing your bed?

Parents are endlessly creative in this area. In my own practice I have talked to a number of co-sleeping fathers and mothers on the subject and written down their responses. Here are a few suggestions I have recorded concerning this issue.

- We put Nicky down early in our bed. When we feel like having sex we do so in the other room.
- My husband got creative on me and rigged a kind of curtain with the crib behind it. When the feeling comes over us we put our newborn into the crib behind the screen and go at it. We are still within earshot of Janice while we do this, but separated by a curtain. Works fine.
- We're not purists. Layla has always had her own room. We put her down to sleep there at bedtime, then when we're ready to go to bed ourselves (and after we have concluded whatever personal business we have together), we carry her in and lay her on a futon next to our bed. We started doing this when she was two years old because she cried so much and begged to sleep with us. We set up this deal, and now she seems perfectly happy with it. No tears or nightmares.
- Since Don still naps, we put him to sleep on the living room couch and go into the bedroom and do our thing. We also get up very early in the morning sometimes and go into another room for sex. If Don cries we hear him. Not perfect, but it's okay for the time being.
- We cheat a little. We put our kid to sleep in one room, then go into another and make love. After a half-hour or however long it takes us, then we bring him back into the bed.

"Like many relational issues," writes McKenna, "parent-child co-sleeping may require unique solutions to assure 'private adult time.' However, that 'problems' in need of solving can be associated with co-sleeping is no more an argument against its legitimacy than is the fact that thousands of parents purchase books to solve the 'problems' associated with solitary infant sleep."[32]

THE NURTURE OF NATURE

When I was a child at camp, I had a cabin counselor who regularly took our group on hikes in the mountains. An amateur botanist and a college student studying zoology, this very special young man would point out the mystical ways of the forest: how buds transform themselves into flowers and then into fruits and berries; how the propeller-shaped seedpods that helicopter down from branches of the maple tree take root and grow into new maple trees; how dead things fall on the spot and fertilize the patch of earth beneath them for years to come; how a vast variety of forest animals eat and are eaten, kill and are killed, in an endless cycle of life and death. He showed us a perpetual ecosystem that functions perfectly on its own without need of improvement or outside help.

One of the most memorable lessons our counselor taught us on those walks was, as he phrased it, "Just let nature take it's course. Nature knows best." When we saw a moth struggling in a web and wanted to free it or when in our destructive male enthusiasm we wanted to dig up a plant or break the branches of a tree, we would hear our counselor's advice and try to follow it as best we could: "Don't disturb it. Just let nature take its course. Nature knows best."

And it does. Of course, there are innumerable instances when technology and scientific advances vastly improve the quality of our health and add to our knowledge of the world—but there are other situations in life, many of them connected to the processes of our own bodies, that are best allowed to unfold on their own according to nature's million-year-old intelligence.

This is especially true of childbirth. In this book we have seen the many ways in which evolution has endowed the human species with a built-in birthing wisdom and a perfectly balanced body ecosystem that needs no improvement or amendment. With the exception of medical abnormalities and birth emergencies, the process of bringing a child into the world operates automatically, like the workings of a fine Swiss watch, helping us, with perfect timing and uncanny precision, to perform on our own—and with the help of trained childbirth professionals—the actions required to bring about a safe, joyous delivery and an enduring bonding period to follow. As so many scientific studies, so many cultural comparisons, so many testimonials, and so many of our own deeper instincts suggest, we tamper with this miraculous mechanism at our peril.

In this chapter, and in this book as a whole, we have discussed some of the most important ways in which we as parents can participate in our newborn's bonding process—encouraging nature and the depthless love it generates between parents and child to take its course.

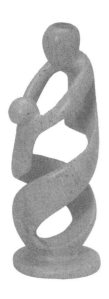

7

The Great Healer

As a society, we have become overwhelmed by this focus on machines and production, so it is not at all surprising that our educational institutions reflect and reinforce this same thinking disorder. As I listen to debates about the so-called oil crisis, it is fascinating (and alarming) to note that all the fixes, from virtually all sides of the political spectrum, focus on production—drill for more oil, build more refineries, create better cars, invent and manufacture new batteries, install sunlight-gathering or wind-harnessing machines, grow more corn, boil hot water, construct nuclear power plants—and so on. And I, working to outgrow this fixation and sensing a crisis of the spirit rather than an energy shortage, keep thinking: reorganize communities, import less stuff, redefine work, share resources, and enhance conviviality. A bit of "pseudo-maximum performance" in these areas and who knows what we might be able to achieve! And promote life learning of the "caring arts" as the single best alternative to ecological devastation.

DAVID ALBERT, EDITOR OF
AND THE SKYLARK SINGS WITH ME NEWSLETTER

The world is hungry. There is a prophecy. It is happening
today: Days are coming . . .
there will be a hunger in the world: but the hunger will
not be for bread and the thirst will not be for water,
but to hear the word of the living G-d.
Everybody believes in G-d, hopefully. But do you know
how much G-d believes in us?
The world still exists. That means G-d believes in us:
believes that we can fix everything.
Let the hungry people get together, you and I, those
hungry to teach our children
One word. Let us get together and fix the world.

RABBI SHLOMO CARLEBACH

THERE IS A SET of questions that is bedeviling American society today. These questions, in a sense, are all one question—a single large and vexing puzzle that can be interpreted in many different ways.

Who is asking this question? Everyone, everywhere.

Pundits are asking it on TV. Films and novels are asking it. You read theories about it in newspapers and magazines and over blogs. You hear it debated by friends at the barbeque, by neighbors over the fence, by coworkers standing together at the office coffee machine. The question is bandied about in the local barbershop and in the nail salon. It is being asked all the time, in every nook and cranny of American society. You cannot escape it, though you cannot always define it. Indeed, from a certain standpoint the question is best expressed in its variations:

Why is there so much violence in our country today? Why do people in this country seem so eager to argue at the drop of a hat, to put others down, to resent, to criticize, to dominate, to fight?

Why are there more people in jail in the United States than in any other country in the industrialized world? Why so many police? Why so many, many laws?

Why are Americans so fearful, disaffected, angry, bottled up and emotionally shut down?

Why do Americans become bored so easily? Why are they so reliant on the stimulation that distracting and mind-numbing entertainments pipe in via TV, movies, video games, popular music, amusement parks, sports? Why do we as a nation seem to be, to invoke the title of a book by NYU professor, Neil Postman, "amusing ourselves to death?"

Why has our traditional sense of community and broad-based family life been replaced by a lonely, isolated kind of independence that is most perfectly symbolized by the image of a single man or a single woman sitting alone in an apartment in front of a TV set with a drink in one hand and a clicker in the other.

Why is there so much mental illness in our country today—depression, paranoia, narcissism, bipolar disorder? Why does one out of five Americans suffer from some form of mental disorder? Why are there so many emotional breakdowns? Why so many psychotic homeless men and women wandering the streets? Why so many suicides? Why so many people living a life of hopeless despair? Why so many criminally insane?

Why are families in America so dysfunctional and split apart? Why do family members, brother and sister, husband and wife, seem so angry at one another so much of the time? Why is there so much violence in families—parents physically and mentally abusing their children, older siblings abusing younger siblings, spouses physically attacking one another? Why are divorces and broken homes so prevalent? Why do so many young people dislike their parents, and why do so many parents dislike their children?

Why are our young people so unhappy and alienated? How, for example, is it possible that children are killing one another on the playground and in school corridors? How is it possible that twelve-year-old girls come to class carrying handguns in their backpacks? How can it be that drug and alcohol abuse, once an affliction suffered exclusively by adults, has infiltrated its way down even to the grade school level of

American schools? Why is there so much meanness and bullying among young people, even between friends? Why are our children so obsessed with sex at such an early age? Why are sexually transmitted diseases so common among adolescents? Why are learning deficits, eating disorders, obesity, depression, hyperactivity, and autism reaching epidemic proportions among the young? Why do five-year-olds and six-year-olds commit the one act that has always been considered unthinkable for a child, and for which there is almost no precedent in the annals of all history: suicide?

The one big question, in other words, the single vast conundrum, is many questions rolled into one, all of which can be boiled down to a single line: *What has gone so very, very wrong with our world?*

~⌒

It would, of course, be far-fetched to imply that this book and the many subjects discussed in it can answer this question.

Or is it far-fetched?

Might it not be said that many of the topics discussed throughout, the case histories, quotes, stories, and scientific findings, all point to a single problem, a single human lack from which so many of the problems that poison society stem?

What exactly is this error?

Let's explore. Let's review where we have come from so far in this book, and in the process inquire after signs and indications that lead us to a greater awareness, both of how to be better parents, and of what is going so terribly wrong in society today.

IN REVIEW

In chapter 1, the irony of this book's title is made painfully clear. The name *The Art of Conscious Parenting* is ironic because the type of birthing and parenting it advocates is as old as humankind and in some ways much older, tracing itself far, far back along the evolving mammalian line. The notion that natural parenting is something new is true only for those who have been brainwashed to believe that technologized childbirth is the only safe, sane way of bringing a child into the world, and that early separation of infants from their mothers makes the child a stronger, better adjusted adult. As mentioned in chapter 1, the new conscious parenting is new, yes—but only to those of us who live a modern Western industrialized way of life.

Throughout this book we have also seen the many dangers inherent in the machine-man paradigm of the human body and of society at large. Equally dangerous is the stealing away of birthing choices from the mother-to-be and the imposed authority of a male-dominated birthing establishment. Indeed, the current model of the delivery room drama is mandated by a hard-and-fast set of rules, which with many possible additions, include the following:

- ❧ Childbirth is a hazardous, unpredictable, and enormously painful procedure.
- ❧ When a woman is with child she is sick. She is suffering from a kind of "disease" and needs to be made well again by removing the foreign object that is growing in her womb.
- ❧ Pregnancy, therefore, is as much a medical condition as, say, a broken leg or a ruptured appendix.

The notion that the expectant mother has birthing instincts, and that she has an innate wisdom concerning how best to deliver her own child (for example, which position to assume during birth, when to push, and so on) is considered a dangerous myth. The gynecologist and obstetrician always know the best procedures during delivery. Despite the mother's emotional wishes and biological intuitions—and sometimes in opposition to them—the doctor is granted total control over the entire process of childbirth as a matter of course and conviction.

High-tech birth demands that a number of electronic machines, some of them invasive, be used to monitor all stages of the pregnant mother's progress; and also, that a pharmacopoeia of chemical medicines be ingested or injected at various stages of pregnancy and birth to help the mother deliver the child in the best possible way. As Robbie Davis-Floyd and Elizabeth Davis tell us, "Basic tenets include the metaphorization of the female body as a defective machine, and the working premise that birth will be 'better' when this defective birthing machine is hooked up to other, more perfect diagnostic machines."[1]

Some form of anesthesia is usually necessary during birth. (In the mid part of the twentieth century it was standard practice to put the expectant mother to sleep before delivery. The mother then woke up hours later with a painful anesthesia hangover, as did her newborn child.)

C-sections are safer than normal delivery and are recommended with increasing frequency by obstetricians. Some doctors even insist that c-sections are the most "organic" form of delivery (just as medical wisdom in the 1940s insisted that baby formula was more nutritious for a newborn than breast milk).

During the entire process of child delivery the mother must assume a motionless, helpless, supine position on the delivery table; and this, despite the fact that it has been known for centuries that squatting or assuming an on-all-fours position is the most effective positions for a fast, easy birth.

Father's have no place in the birthing room. They are advised to wait patiently outside the delivery room while the medical professionals do the job.

To this list, add the many strange, unnecessary, and sometimes injurious practices that are routinely applied in the delivery chamber: early cutting of the umbilical cord and the consequent danger to the newborn of oxygen deprivation and brain damage; random use of chemicals such as oxytocin to induce labor; fetal monitoring. We could mention many more of the unnatural ways that modern obstetrics has changed the age-old rhythms and practices of childbirth, and turned what should be a parent's proudest moment into a dark journey through an anxious and inhospitable high-tech hospital maze.

And what is the result of all this tampering with nature?

How do these practices affect the newborn child and the grownup person this child someday becomes? What is the result of technologized pregnancy and birth, and an infancy lived in isolation from the parents? An infancy spent sleeping in a separate room? An infancy ruled by Dr. Spock's dictum to ignore the nighttime cries of the child? An infancy where the mother is habitually absent from the child? An infancy lived out in daycare? An infancy watched over by a revolving door of babysitters? An infancy where touching, playing, caressing, rubbing, massaging, and affection between mother and child are in short supply?

What does this all add up to in terms of early childhood growth and later adult development? What kind of children does our present system of childbirth and early child rearing produce when parents have been marginalized?

BREAKING THROUGH AND BREAKING UP

One of the foremost leaders in the field of early child development, Dr. James Prescott, was born during the Great Depression in America. His parents died at an early age, and Dr. Prescott, along with his three brothers, was left orphaned and forced to spend a majority of his childhood deprived of a normal family structure.

Needless to say, this deprivation left a searing impression on Dr. Prescott's mind. Yet eventually it was to become a positive force in his life, guiding him to a choice of academic career where he could study early childhood development and the effect that absence of parental love had on infants.

In 1966, Dr. Prescott joined the newly formed National Institute of Child Health and Human Development (NICHD). Here he formed the Developmental Behavioral Biology Program and became its Health Scientist Administrator, a post that he held until 1980.

As mandated by the NICHD, Dr. Prescott's task was to conduct "research and training in the special health problems and requirements of mothers and children." The principal intent of his investigations was to use scientific methods to better understand the relationship between early mother-child separation and its possible links to violence, suicide, crime, and depression in the adult population.

During his fourteen-year stay at the NICHD, Dr. Prescott and his associates concentrated much of their attention on abuse of the parent-child relationship. Following the instructions to the NICHD of then Secretary of the Department of Education and Welfare, Casper Weinberger, to "expand its studies to uncover the origins of child abuse and neglect and of violence in the home," Prescott's team came up with many groundbreaking and startling discoveries. Foremost among them was that failed bonding between a mother and her infant child can trigger measurable biochemical brain changes in a child and resultant mental disorders. In adult life these disorders could then lead to many miseries: depression, anxiety, eating disorders, drug abuse, addiction, violence, criminal activity, psychosis, and suicide.

What types of behavior on the part of the mother, according to Dr. Prescott's findings, actually lead to failed bonding? The following is a partial list:

- Lack of caressing and loving touch bestowed on infants by parents, and especially by the mother
- Frequent harsh scolding and discipline
- Lack of intimate, loving play between mother/father and infant
- Chronic lack of attention paid to the infant by the mother
- Continual and prolonged separations between mother and child
- A cold, aloof, loveless, and indifferent attitude toward the child
- Physical abuse of any kind

There are more items that fit the list. You can probably add a few yourself. But at the same time, there is also a set of affirmative maternal behaviors that lead to a successful and bonded mother-child relationship. For example:

- ∮ The parents constantly touch and fondle the infant (massaging, caressing, kissing, hugging).
- ∮ There is frequent eye contact between mother and child. The mother smiles often and lovingly at the child. Mother and child laugh together frequently.
- ∮ Parents and child play together constantly, tickling, making faces, stroking.

(I tickle, wrestle, make faces, tell jokes, snuggle, and say prayers every night with my ten-year-old son and always kiss him goodnight. We call it kibitz-time.)

Holding up colorful images, crawling on the floor together, listening to music, rolling balls, arranging blocks and shapes works well for little ones.

- ∮ The mother talks constantly to the child in a warm, intimate voice, often whispering loving words in his or her ear.
- ∮ Mother and child are constantly together, preferably making skin-to-skin contact via a sling or child-carrying device.
- ∮ The child is breastfed for at least one year and preferably two or more.

In its time, during the 1970s, these and other findings that Dr. Prescott and his colleagues came up with exerted a marked influence on the way to mental health. Professionals began to look—and relook—at the maternal bond. New light was shone on age-old human problems. Reassessments were made. New techniques were devised for raising children without trauma or conflict. Many of the troubles that beset the human race, it seemed, were biologically induced by parents. What's more, the brain chemistry imbalance caused by lack of maternal con-nection could be avoided and even repaired. How? Simply by loving the child, always and everywhere. By bonding.

Here, it seemed, was a powerful key to solving the mysteries of human violence and despair. Here was something unique, something measurable and scientific, something that promised to set us on a sane new course that would change our world.

Imagine, then, the dark cloud that passed over the initial jubila-tion in the child development community when, in 1980, the NICHD did a sudden reversal, insisting, in the words of agency head, Norman Kretchmer that "we were never in child abuse or domestic violence research. Our work is in the area of child development."

Despite protests, despite resistance from members of Congress, despite the outcry of the psychiatric community, despite the existence of records specifically mandating that the NICHD perform research in the field of maternal deprivation and abuse, Dr. Prescott's program was cancelled, his job was terminated, and almost all the records pertaining to his work were destroyed.

GOING IT ON YOUR OWN

It is beyond the scope of this book to unravel the highly politicized reasons behind this abrupt and, in the eyes of many child development workers, tragic reversal of policy by the NICHD. There is, however, something profoundly important for us to note in this cautionary tale of sound science and useful applied psychology nipped in the bud.

And this something is as follows: in a society where special interests, especially profit-driven medical and pharmaceutical special interests, exert such a profound influence over laws and social policies, it is dif-ficult for progressive work in child development to receive the attention, funding, and sympathy it so obviously deserves.

Equally important for our purposes is the fact that these special-interest groups are dedicated to making sure that the current status quo is neither challenged nor changed, and that our government, so often under the sway of big money concerns, will do little in the future to change its educational and medical standards for the rearing of children in our society.

Given this situation, it thus becomes the task of all of us, of you and me, of each individual person, to take the bull by the horns and apply the principles of the new parenting on our own.

For the fact is that there *is* support and guidance in these areas if you seek it. There are like-minded people, doctors and nurses among them, who are sympathetic to the ideas of The New Conscious Parenting, and who will help you take the first steps toward natural child rearing, with all the empowering techniques that are part of it.

In chapter 2, I described the amazing journey my wife, Dalit, and I took, first in finding a sympathetic and informed childbirthing professional to deliver our child, and second, in making full use of a hospital birthing center to deliver our son in the easiest, least painful, most satisfying, and yes, beatific way possible.

Ten years have now passed since the day of Kesem's birth, and I see with the eye of a trained professional that my son is growing up strong and confident, sensitive, alert, and kind. He mixes well with others. He enjoys the company of all kinds of people. He is self-possessed, friendly, unprejudiced, and most of all fearless, standing unafraid in the face of schoolyard bullies, new situations, things that go bump in the night, and all the terrors of abandonment and loneliness that scar so many childhoods. Intellectually he is inquisitive and insightful. He reads a great deal, enjoys music of all kinds, and lives in his own world of creative imagination. Emotionally he is affectionate, confident, cheerful, and always willing to give another person the benefit of the doubt.

Why is Kesem so well adjusted? Good genes? Perhaps to some small extent, but probably not to the degree that is commonly supposed.

In fact, Kesem's positive maturity is, I believe, due largely to the fact that we as informed parents bucked conventional wisdom and adopted an educational model based on the ideas presented in this book, a model that places parent-child love, respect, true information, and bonding above all other concerns. *Always with unconditional love.* Not for what you do (for me) but for who you are in your being. Not through rewards and punishments but through love and *reason.* Knowing the *needs* of the child before he does, and giving what's necessary, will take care of 90 percent of your parenting. Being a bonded parent gives you an intuitive sense, an inner knowing, which unbonded parents do not have. This means if your child does something bad, you inform him that it is not acceptable behavior. But you still give him love. You do not punish by withholding love or abandon him to teach him a lesson. You will most likely have to repeat this reason over and over again. Children absorb only through repetition. And repetition is the mother of skill. It is through the social and behavioral skills that your child will become a successful adult. Most of the damaged adults I see in my practice need to be taught the life skills they never got when they were little children.

There is, I should say, nothing special about my wife and me. We are like any other parents who wish the best for their child. We guided our son down the path of sanity and wholeness, I believe, first because we were informed on the subject of natural child-raising, having read the work of Joseph Chilton Pearce, Bruce Lipton, James Prescott, Suzanne Arms, Michel Odent, Robbie Davis-Floyd, and other child-development specialists whose voices you have heard throughout this book. Second, because we talked to everyone we knew who had knowledge of natural child-development procedures: doctors, midwives, psychologists, assorted health care professionals, and other parents. Finally, because we persisted, taking the knowledge and skills developed by so many brilliant thinkers, and applying them to the raising of our own son. As our son matures and becomes a teen, I am sure that these conscious-parenting techniques will continue to be successful.

Thus, at risk of sounding like a too proud parent, I am going to take a few pages to describe some of the specific techniques my wife and I used to bond with our son.

I include these descriptions, I should say, not to toot our horn, but to provide a model that other parents can use and that will help guide them along the very difficult path of child raising. As one of my patients remarked when her six-year-old daughter was caught in school with a pack of cigarettes in her knapsack, "You have to be the Buddha to raise a sane kid in this society!"

I agree.

SPEAKING FIRST HAND

When Kesem was a newborn child, Dalit made certain to take him with her wherever she went. During their time out of the house, Dalit carried Kesem pressed tightly against her body in a sling, but with Kesem's head positioned high enough so that he could make eye contact with passing strangers and observe the bustling world around him—this, rather than lying flat on his back in a stroller, staring up at a blank sky or at the looming trunks of men and women moving by him like lampposts seen from a car window.

"I used to always carry Kesem in a baby carrier wherever I went during the day," Dalit told me in a taped interview I made for this book. "I'd take him everywhere—*everywhere*. On the bus, shopping, to the library, visiting friends, the mall. Everywhere."

From Dalit's perspective, any social encounter was an opportunity to develop her son's heart and mind.

When she and Kesem went shopping at the grocery store, for example, she would turn this ordinary event into a finely tuned learning experience. "When we walked down the aisles of the supermarket," she says, "I'd say to Kesem, 'Look, this is an apple,' and I'd hold it up in front of him. 'See, this is a pear. This is a vegetable. A carrot. A head of lettuce.' I'd show him all the forms of food, all the colors. He'd watch me put the beets into the plastic bag and weigh them. I'd hold a fresh peach up to him and let him smell it, touch it. I'd let him run peanuts in the shell through his fingers."

As a conscious parenting mother, Dalit held tight to the notion that it is never too early to introduce abstract thinking to a child.

"When we got near the checkout counter, I'd talk to Kesem about the price of the groceries, and introduce the concept of numbers and math. I'd say, 'Here, this box of salt, it costs one dollar. This bottle of oil, it costs three dollars.

"Then I'd show him what a dollar bill looks like as I paid for the groceries. He'd just sit there in his baby sling listening attentively to everything I said. Sometimes he'd reach out to touch one of the objects, or just start to giggle. He was clearly gobbling up impressions and enjoying himself immensely. He was, you could say, totally engaged instead of lying there like baggage at the bottom of a baby carriage. All his mind and senses and feelings were being used to the fullest, and he liked it. Loved it. All babies do."

What's interesting to note is that when Dalit toted Kesem and the two set out on their daily rounds, they frequently found themselves in overcrowded spaces or walking down loud, busy streets. But this noise and clamor was stimulating to Kesem rather than intimidating. He never cried when he was in chaotic situations but remained placid and alert, much in the vein, you will recall, of the contented infants Marcelle Geber saw while studying birthing practices in Uganda.

Why did Kesem cry so seldom? Because he was exactly were he should be, pressed tight against his mother in a warm, safe, protected environment. This is what all infants want, along with food and dry diapers: maternal security.

"I was always there for him," Dalit says. "From the day we came home from the hospital I was there with him to meet his needs. Kids only cry because their cues and their needs—the need to be changed, let's say, or paid attention to, to be fed—are not met. So they start crying. Seems obvious. But if the mother is there for them ready to attend to all their needs there's no cause for fuss. They can spend the time instead looking around and getting to know the world."

∽

There are two primary drives hard-wired into every child. The first is to feel safe and bonded with the mother. After that need is met, the energy of the child is free to go to the second drive, which is to explore the world. If the first need is not met, the child feels anxiety. This takes away the energy to explore his world, and thus his ability to learn is hampered. He will learn anyway, but not as well.

This is not to say you must be perfect to be a good parent. You can make mistakes and your child will still be okay. It is in the *intention* to use the art and science of conscious parenting and the bond of love with your child that at the end of the day will work for you both.

The infant child's education, needless to say, is not exclusive to the outside world. It can go on with the same intensity while at home. "We never childproofed our house," Dalit relates. "Instead, we educated Kesem at a very early age about the objects in the house and which things he should be careful of. Instead of the 'Don't touch, don't touch, no, no, no!' bit all the time, we'd explain to him what everything was, in simple, plain, matter-of-fact English.

"For instance, we took him on a tour of our home many times. We showed him the furnishings and said, 'Here, feel this.' If we had a porcelain globe we'd hand it to him and tell him, 'See, this is pottery, now touch it, feel it, tap on it.' If a surface was clean we'd let him place his mouth on it and taste it, as taste is such a primary tool for an infant's education. Or if there was a metal object we'd rap on it so he could hear its particular sound, and later he could make the connection between this sound and all things made of metal. In other words, we explained things to him rather than scolding him or making him fearful."

Jean Leidloff is author of the book *Continuum Concept,* a famous study based on her observations of parenting practices among members of the Yequana tribe in Venezuela. After spending a good deal of time recording the benevolent ways in which Yequana mothers educate their children, she had this to say about teaching appropriate childhood behaviors.

We should never do anything to a child that will make him feel badly about himself. But we do this all the time. We do it with words and we do it with looks. We only know two ways to treat our children. One is punishing/blaming: "you are very bad, go stand in the corner or I'll spank you." The other is permissive: "that's perfectly all right darling, if you want to walk on mother's face, she doesn't mind." We don't know any other way.[2]

According to Liedloff, there is, in fact, a third way.

It is called information. If you thoroughly understand that children are innately social, then you understand that what they want is information. You don't have to be angry to tell them what's needed. You just let them know. The idea is not to blame, and not to praise, because both can be insulting. Expect children to do the right thing. You then are being a clear model and there's no conflict. It's the way nature designed us to behave.[3]

Taking a lead from Liedloff, we applied her ideas when teaching Kesem the principles of household safety. Again, infants are much more receptive to instruction than most parents suppose. The key is repetition—giving reasonable explanations to a child over and over again until the message sinks in.

"We introduced him to the idea that glass can break," Dalit says. "Then we'd take an old glass from the kitchen and a high-sided metal box. We'd say, 'Now don't get scared, it's okay,' and we would drop the glass into the box and watch it break into a bunch of pieces. Kesem got a little upset at first when we did this but we said, 'No, that's okay. That's how it works. We want you to understand that glass can break. Metal feels like this and looks like this, but it doesn't break. Glass does.' And so forth.

"Then we'd do the same with knives. Whenever I cooked Kesem was always with me in the kitchen. I'd put him in a highchair at counter level so he could look at what I was doing. When I was cutting food with a sharp knife I'd give him a plastic knife and let him cut a big cucumber or a soft banana for himself. So that he felt like he was participating in family chores, and that he was capable of doing grownup things. While I was showing him how to cut I'd point to the blade on my knife, and tell that this is sharp, do not touch it. 'Never touch a blade,' I'd say. 'It's sharp.' I would put that kind of emphasis on it. I wouldn't say 'No, no, it's bad!' I would say 'Sharp' or 'Dangerous, be careful!' I'd just tell him the facts, and let him take it from there." I would still be quite careful, however, even though you are educating your child. That does not make it okay to leave sharp knives lying on the coffee table."

Understand that while Dalit was taking Kesem through many of these learning calisthenics, he was still an infant. Many parents assume that because very young children do not communicate with spoken language they are incapable of making logical deductions, recognizing differences and contrasts, remembering what they see, drawing relationships between objects, and so forth.

In fact, quite the opposite is true: Children are never more susceptible to empirical learning than they are in the months following birth. At this point in their development, both their senses and their unconscious minds are wide open, totally susceptible to whatever sounds and sights are taken in. "Just as it took nature nine months to grow that infant in the mother's womb," writes Joseph Chilton Pearce, "it takes another nine months 'in arms' to firmly establish that infant in the matrix of the new world."[4]

New parenting mothers and fathers are well advised to take advantage of this openness, and to turn the circumstances of ordinary life into a living schoolroom. This opportunity is golden and precious. Once it has passed it never returns. Seize the opportunity!

"Sometimes we would go to the post office," Dalit continues. "I'd show Kesem the letters, the stamps. I'd mail a letter and tell him it was going to his grandmother in Israel, or to pay a bill—numbers again.

We'd look at all the people coming into the post office and going out. I'd describe the scene for him, point out the things people were wearing and the objects they were holding: that lady over there is carrying a brown purse, this boy here has a big yellow package in his hands. I'd describe when people were smiling, when they were laughing, talking, paying for things, whatever, all to give him a general sense of the human give-and-take that occurs in a social setting."

Also instrumental to Kesem's education was contact with nature.

Even if you live in a big city there is almost always enough green somewhere to provide contact with the organic world. A local park, an empty lot, a tree on a tree-lined street, a grassy patch by the side of the road, all can quickly be turned into a learning laboratory for the infant mind. "I'd take Kesem to the city park every day," Dalit says. "We'd sit on the ground together and play with the soil. I'd bring a little spoon and some digging toys. I'd dig into the earth and I'd show him worms. I would show him soil. And let him get dirty. See it and smell it. I'd let him walk barefooted. Or we'd roll on the grass together. I'd give him a flower to play with or a piece of bark, a handful of pebbles. We'd pick dandelions and study them up close. Children at this age need very little to introduce them to the natural environment.

"Sometime we'd all travel as a family too, to some lovely spot outside the city, to a river or a state park. Kesem loved all these trips at the earliest age. All kids love nature outings; they love nature instinctively. The same way they love animals. It's part of their makeup as human beings. They share the planet with other living creatures, and somehow they're aware of this fact from the very start.

"So I would take advantage of this fact and bring him into contact with rocks, sand, water, trees, let him feel their texture, and smell them, and play with them. I'd point out the animals like squirrels and dogs. We'd feed the pigeons. To this day, Kesem loves to just sit in the park and watch the birds or to play games with a few leaves and some grass and stones."

When Kesem was old enough to interact with other children, the park now served as a get-to-know-you center and as an instruction manual in social interactivity.

"When he was three or four I'd take him by the hand to give him a totally secure feeling. Give him the feeling that absolutely everything is going to be okay when he sees the other kids, because I'm right here, holding his hand, and I'm here talking to the mothers, and I'm here talking to the other children. I wanted him to experience the feeling of being included. I would go from park to park, bringing him up to the children. I'd tell him to introduce himself and to say, 'Hi, my name is Kesem. Can I play with you? Can I play ball with you? Can I ride the bicycle with you? Can we jump together in the pool? Can you throw the ball to me?' The other kids always said, 'Okay.'"

"Slowly, we worked on it, week after week, and he'd do exactly what I told him to do. After a while he was able to go into any new environment, even if it was filled with total strangers and introduce himself. Before long he would be playing with these strange kids as if they were his oldest friends. Sometimes he'd become the leader, telling kids older than himself what games to play. At eight years old, Kesem was totally at ease with children his own age and with adults. He makes conversation easily, he introduces himself to new people, he listens to what others say and makes intelligent responses. I can't help but think that all those interactions he had with other people as a very young child served as a kind of training grounds for the social skills he shows today."

Stores and places of business, Dalit notes, are excellent places for teaching children the rules of social exchange. "I'd take him into a bank or retail store. I'd tell him that it was okay to laugh in these stores. He could sing here, he could make faces. I would put him up on the counter at the bank while I was depositing money. They never see kids in a bank, you know. The kids are either at day care or at school or below eye level in a stroller. So after a while the tellers would get to know Kesem and then make him their mascot. They looked forward to him coming, and as time went on he developed different relationships with different tellers. It was all the beginning of learning the social graces."

What was most important about these interactions with adults was that they encouraged Kesem to feel he was as important as grownups are, even though he was so young. That he mattered, that he had the respect and interest of other people, and that he wasn't just a piece of furniture.

"I didn't want Kesem to feel that he was somehow inferior to grownups just because he was pint-sized. Some parents, you see them always telling their kids how little or helpless they are. This, I think, makes children feel fragile and unsafe all the time. Like something terrible is going to happen to them because they're so small. We as parents tried to do the opposite. We tried to empower Kesem. To make him feel that he was the equal—not the better, but the equal—of anyone he met."

I myself remember a significant incident that took place when Kesem was two-and-a-half years old. Dalit and I brought him into a jewelry store. Standing behind the counter was a sophisticated sales lady. She had lots of makeup and jewelry on. Expensive clothes. The woman came over to Kesem and exclaimed, "What an adorable little boy, how cute! Can I give you a kiss?"

Kesem looked back at her for a long moment, then simply said, "No."

The woman was taken aback and looked up at us, as if we were supposed to tell him how rude he was, and then *make* him kiss the woman. But we weren't having any of it. Dalit simply shrugged at the sales lady and said, "He doesn't want you to kiss him."

Then we walked out of the store.

BOILING FROGS

There is a story I have often heard. I cannot vouch for its scientific accuracy, as I have never tried to boil a frog. What is most interesting to me about this story is the metaphor it draws.

Take a frog, the story goes, and drop it into a vat of boiling water. Immediately the frog will panic and leap out of the pot.

Now try another tactic. Place the frog into a vat of cool water. Then *very* gradually turn up the heat. Amazingly (as the scenario goes), the frog will sit there dumbly and allow the heat to consume it.

Why? Because the heat comes on so slowly, so imperceptibly that the frog does not notice it—until, finally, its powers are spent and it is too weak to escape.

What's significant about this story for our concerns is the tie that can be made between the process of animal conditioning and society's current woes. The idea is this: if harmful influences are introduced into a culture in a gradual way over an extended period of time—influences that weaken the culture and that deprive its citizens of their personal and biological rights—they too, like the frog, will fail to notice what is being done to them until it is too late.

The changes we are talking about have been occurring over the centuries, perhaps even since the era of the Industrial Revolution. This slow transformation from agrarian to urban, hand-made to mass-produced, cooperative to competitive, religious to secular, natural to chemical, plastic, and electronic, have ushered in many new paradigms including all the usual suspects: exploitation of the environment, destruction of species, overpopulation, pollution of the air and water, wars fought over natural resources, fragmenting of the nuclear family, the corporate drive for monetary profit at all costs, and many more.

As time passes, and as these new paradigms replace the old, traditional wisdoms, the generations that follow know little of the truths that their parents and grandparents once took for granted. Until one day the world is qualitatively different from what it had once been; and so are the people in it.

All this, needless to say, is not new news. We have heard these matters discussed many times over the years; and, it should be said, there are encouraging signs that people are discovering what has been stolen from them by the corporate techno-state, and are making attempts on many levels to retrieve their lost values.

For our purpose, however, there is one loss in particular that is more devastating than all the others, and which is, in a sense, responsible for them. This loss, as James Prescott and other enlightened child-development professionals tell us, causes most of the problems outlined at the beginning of this chapter.

And this one loss is, in a word, the loss of *bonding*.

Bonding, with all that the word implies: closeness, accord, unity, compassion, cooperation, forbearance, human touch, mutual love, maternal affection. Or conversely, loss of bonding: to be frightened, fragmented, lonely, suspicious, untrusting, cut off, and separate from other people. To believe that survival can only be accomplished by conquering others. By accumulating more money and material goods than everyone else. By taking care of number one at the exclusion of all else.

The loss of bonding between mother and child, between people everywhere, and between nations of the world is, I believe, the primary cause of the violence and alienation that is so endemic to our times. As the saying goes: "Take away heat, and you have cold. Take away love and you have hate." For in the big picture, bonding is produced by love. My working definition of love: Love is not simply a feeling. It is not just an idea or an attraction or a sensation. Love is a particular kind of irradiation that is generated by one person and received by another. It can only occur through an *action* with the *intention* of helping and caring for the other.

If I am too busy to help you there is no irradiation, no love. If I come to your aid in spite of the fact that I'm angry or annoyed with you, this is love. And an irradiation is given and received. And this is bonding too.

An example: A husband asks his wife, "Darling, would you close the window? I'm cold."

If she answers, "What am I, your slave?" There is no love here, and consequently no irradiation given off. So no bonding takes place.

But if she happily closes the window, this act becomes a loving act, and an irradiation is given, received, and ultimately reciprocated. And the window has nothing to do with it. It is the *action* with the *intention* of helping.

This give-and-take of caring energy between people can take place, and should take place, not only with parent and child, friend and friend, but with pets as well, and even with plants. Every living organism wants and needs love. Without it the world withers. With it all is well. In this light the claim of Ralph Waldo Emerson that "we make all our own heaven, and we make our own hell" takes on new meaning.

In regard to the universal need for bonding, Joseph Chilton Pearce is once again devastatingly articulate in describing the ways in which loss of love and bonding affects every tier of human society, as well as every level of the human psyche.

Is bonding all that important? . . . James W. Prescott's theoretical and scientific research on the origins of love and violence cuts to the core of our personal and global violence. The closer we come to the source of our pain, however, the more we tend to defend against it, a response that often blinds us to the obvious.

Human love begins *in utero,* is carried through pregnancy, birth, and the postnatal nurturance of bonding and breast-feeding. Yet, the most critical, formal relationship—one that encodes the developing brain for a lifetime of affection or rage—the relationship between the mother and infant, is not valued, nurtured, or supported by our culture. Infants and young children are often not held, touched, or played with. The majority of babies are placed in institutional-ized childcare. Television and computers have replaced imaginative play between adults and children. Failing the early bond, which is intimately linked to direct and sustained physical contact between mother and infant, the future of later love relationships is threat-ened, as is society itself. Unbonded behavior results in an alienated, aggressive emotional/social/sexual cycle that affects mother, baby, family, society, and now the world.[5]

The process of creating an unbonded human being, as we have seen in many examples, begins at birth. The moment a child emerges from the womb he or she is removed from the mother. This separation becomes emblematic of the modern parent-child relationship that will follow. It continues into infancy where many societal forces impinge on families, forcing them, often against their will, to give a child up to state or private sponsored daycare or educational facilities where they languish far from the nurturance and loving education of their rightful teachers—their parents.

Soon the forces of separation take over entirely. Children in daycare. Children alone in front of the TV. Children playing endless video games and surfing the Net. Children left in a room alone at night to cry themselves to sleep. Children four and five years old confined to a school room for an entire day, staring at computer screens, punished for nonconformity, deprived of the hour-to-hour bonding exchanges that parents know in their hearts are the natural order of a child's well-being.

And what, in the long run, is the result of all these deprivations?

A broken world.

TIKKUN

The circle completes itself, and we return to the basic idea mentioned in chapter 2: fixing the world. Tikkun is Hebrew for rectification or fixing, and used in this exact context; fixing the world.

Surely, it is clear by now that we cannot rely on our leaders and our governments and our politicians and our corporations to set things straight in the world. These people and institutions are largely responsible for causing the problems in the first place.

No, the act of "fixing the world," of transforming our planet from a violent, selfish, exploitive place into a "city of love," one relies on individual initiative, and on the collective efforts that people make when they come together, share constructive and progressive ideas, and put these ideas into practice.

For example, every time we perform a kindly act for our child, for a friend, for a stranger, the bond between hearts and minds among all people everywhere is strengthened. Every time we are cruel or uncaring, the forces of separation prevail. It all begins and ends on an individual level: with you and with me. "No man is an island entire of itself," writes the British poet, John Donne, in "Meditation 17." "Every man is a piece of the continent, a part of the main. If a clod is washed away by the sea, Europe is the less . . . any man's death diminishes me, because I am involved in mankind, and therefore never ask to know for whom the bell tolls; it tolls for thee." (In eighteenth-century England they rang a bell when someone died.)

What then are the specific things we can do to produce physically and mentally healthy children who will go into the world and make it a better place?

Start with education. Read everything you can on the subjects mentioned throughout this book. Learn the options. Talk to people who have used natural birthing and natural educational techniques with their own child. Subscribe to nonviolent magazines and periodicals. Get on blog lists for natural parenting. Place yourself in the mainstream of new parenting thinking. Get to know it. Then put what you've learned into practice.

For pregnant couples, consider meeting with a nurse midwife. See if you feel comfortable. Talk to her about the possibility of a delivery at a natural birthing center and what that would be like using the services of a midwife. Take a natural birthing class. During the birth, and even before, parents can apply the many bonding techniques described throughout this book. Once home, the bonding then continues for years to come, with parents and child eating together, sleeping together, traveling together, playing together, praying together, enjoying each other's company, and learning from each other's innate wisdoms. It is all simply a question of learning, then doing.

There is a fairy story I heard once when I was a small boy, and it has stayed with me ever since: Once long ago, the story tells, there was a young tree living in a large, lush green forest. All the trees in this forest loved one another, and this love transformed their forest into a place of happiness and light.

Then one day a woodsman came to the forest and chopped down the young tree. When this happened a great sadness filled the forest, and the trees in the great forest began to wilt.

The young tree, meanwhile, was transported to a large city where skillful hands sliced it into pieces and used its wood to build a violin.

This violin is still being played to this day, the story goes, and its melodies are filled with a sad yearning—a yearning to return to the forest, to live again among the trees, to be part of the community of trees.

And isn't it true that sometimes we ourselves also hear this sad melody? Doesn't its sound remind us of our own separation from the center, and of the deep longing we all harbor, deep inside us beneath all the cares and turmoil of ordinary life, to be united in loving concord with others of our kind—and thus with all being and creation?

This concord is, I believe, the treasure that is waiting to be claimed by people who are courageous enough and far-seeing enough and wise enough to practice the new parenting.

Onward and upward.

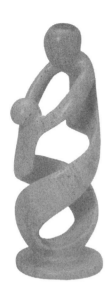

Thinking of Conscious Parenting as Green Parenting

BECAUSE IN THIS DAY and age when the world is going green, and when so many of us are concerned with energy conservation and all the ramifications of ecological balance and economic cost controls, following the suggestions in *The Art of Conscious Parenting* will not only save parents energy and money, but billions of wasted dollars in future medical expenses and lost hours of work due to depression, addictions, and broken homes. By treating children with the love and respect they so desperately need, parents automatically help defer the cost of the human "unbonded." That is, they stop the process of putting unthinkably expensive bandages on worldwide problems, and in its place they apply the simple teachings presented in this book—teachings that provide the ounce of prevention humanity so dearly needs today.

As we have said in the last chapter; unbonded people create a broken world. Our planet is a living being. Where there is movement there is life. Where the part is alive, the whole is alive. This Earth is our mother. Like a huge breast she nurtures the thin film of organic life that thrives on her surface. We, in turn, are her caretakers. Our mother's womb is our first matrix where we form our body, senses, and perceptions, and where we prepare for our entry into the second matrix: Mother. It is here in this all important second matrix in which we develop, or do not develop the skills we will need in the third matrix: World. If we have no bond to our individual mother how can we begin to have a perception of a global mother as well?

Regrettably, the high-tech post-modern industrial cultures that have created so many of the ecological problems that face us today are blind to the aliveness of this world; blind to the enormous damage we are causing to our Mother's ecosystems balance. But take heart: there is a true planetary awakening taking place all around us, one that gives us hope that a real re-greening of the world is unfolding. And happily, the art of conscious parenting is part of this process.

In his classic book, *The Last Hours of Ancient Sunlight,* Thom Hartmann explores the world's population explosion. He shows how cultures and species are being methodically wiped out in every part of the biosphere, and how we have already reached the halfway point of our supplies of petroleum. Humans the world over, he maintains, are facing a crisis of choice in how to create a sustainable future. He proposes that the only lasting solution to the crisis is to relearn the lessons our ancient ancestors knew so well.

They lived a "spiritual ecology" with a view of the sacred nature of *all* creation. They practiced the respect for the living earth and transmitted this to each generation through sacred and intentional rituals. Rupert Sheldrake in his incredible book *The New Science of Life* has scientifically demonstrated that there is a "morphic field" wherein we are all connected. Carl Jung referred to a similar concept as the "collective unconscious."

Hartmann speaks of the thousands of people, today, who are forming a new generation of "tribes"—small intentional communities where people care for each other and live in a sustainable way. And for this it is not necessary to form these communities as physical communal living. They are communities of light, the light of shared vision of the transformation of this planet. Today we can meet with like-minded people in virtual space on the Web. Join conscious circles of learning how to redeem this world.

We have lost our freedom to the "slavery" of civilization. By reconnecting to the wisdom of our ancient ancestors we can learn to touch the sacred. Hartmann goes on:

We can learn the secret of "enough" and how to look into the eyes of God. How? His mentor, Gottfried Muller, told him, "Look into the eyes of any other living thing, there, in the eyes of a cat or a dog, in the eyes of a fly or fish or the eyes of a friend or enemy, and you are looking into the eyes of God."

Most of the ancient peoples lived as a tribe. The most basic unit of the tribe is the family. Many tribes are comprised of a single extended family, often only a dozen people. In America the most well-known tribe is the Kennedys. They have a sense of "this is us" among them. Many people today have chosen to sacrifice family culture and the importance of being together to build a sense of shared experience, for the culture of consumerism. Again, here, the good news is that millions of people are choosing to redirect their time and energy to their family—in a very real sense, their own tribe.

The world is beginning to embrace the need for *sustainability*. As a result, conscious parenting is a guarantor for your children and mine, that they will help to create a living and self-sustaining world. Hartmann states:

While most city-state civilizations throughout history have self-destructed; at least one, the Hebrews (which is actually a tribal nation that is also a city-state civilization) have survived and are the only ones to regain their original ancient lands. While nobody still worships the gods of the Sumarians, Greeks, or Romans—their civilizations are gone—the deity of the Hebrews is still worshipped, in one way or another, by the billions of members of the three major religions of the world. [Author's thought: The world needs religion. However, in the original sense of the word, which comes from the

Latin: *relegere. Legere* is the root word for ligament. *Religion, then, is to be rebound to the source of our being.*]

The ancient Jews were called upon to build into their code of civilization a set of checks and balances called *Sabbath*, the *Shmita*, and the *Jubilee*. Most people know of the Sabbath day, a day of physical rest and spiritual renewal. However, in the Old Testament, the Torah, the concept was carried much further. Every seventh year (Shmita) the land was required to have a Sabbath, too, and no crops could be grown or harvested in that year. (This ritual, plus other aspects of it, is practiced today by many in Israel.) Those fruits that grow on their own are to be left for the poor. This allows the land to rest and recover its fertility, provides a basis for sustainable agriculture, and takes care of the poor.

The Jubilee was an institution of biblical law providing every fifty years for the release of Hebrew slaves, the forgiving of debt, and the restoration of family property. The laws of the Jubilee enabled every Jew in the tribe to begin life again on an equal basis. These and many other lessons from our ancient ancestors allowed them to live sustainably for hundreds and thousands of years without doing a modicum of damage to the earth they loved so much.

The teachings of *The Art of Conscious Parenting* are thus "Green Parenting." They espouse a way of life that "does no harm," that provides the raw materials of a happy, healthy existence, that protects our health rather than undermines it, and that provides for the transmission of these ideas and intentional rituals to endow future generations with the ability to "think with the heart and feel with the brain." Most of all, the teachings of *The Art of Conscious Parenting* champion a realization that the connectivity of all life begins with the mother and with the nuclear family. Our most precious gift in this world is our family—our family *and* the earth, which give us life.

Notes

CHAPTER 1.
A NEW—OR OLD—WAY TO THINK ABOUT BIRTH

1. James W. Prescott, *The Origins of Love & Violence,* DVD from the author.

CHAPTER 2.
HIGH-TECH BIRTH AND THE ALTERNATIVE

1. Robbie Davis-Floyd, *Birth as an American Rite of Passage* (Berkeley: University of California Press, 1992).
2. Ibid.
3. Ibid.
4. Robbie Davis-Floyd and Carolyn Sargeant, *Childbirth and Authoritative Knowledge: Cross-Cultural Perspectives* (Berkeley: University of California Press, 1997).
5. Ibid.
6. Michel Odent, *The Caesarean* (London: Free Association Books, 2004). Most of the facts presented in this section are taken from chapters 4, 5, and 6.
7. Brigitte Jordan, *Birth in Four Cultures: A Cross-Cultural Investigation of Childbirth in Yucatan, Holland, Sweden, and the United States* (Prospect Heights, Ill.: Waveland Press, 1993).
8. Ibid.
9. Ibid.
10. Ibid.
11. Ibid.
12. Ibid.

13. Joseph Chilton Pearce, *Magical Child* (New York: Plume, 1992).

14. Ibid.

15. Ibid.

16. Ibid.

17. Meredith F. Small, *Our Babies, Ourselves* (New York: First Anchor Books, 1999).

18. Ibid.

19. Dr. William Sears and Martha Sears, *The Baby Book* (Boston: Little Brown, 1992).

20. Joseph Chilton Pearce, *Magical Child,* 51.

21. Michel Odent, *The Caesarean,* 24.

22. Ibid.

23. Joseph Chilton Pearce, *Magical Child.*

CHAPTER 3. A CHILD'S FIRST SCHOOLHOUSE: LEARNING IN THE WOMB

1. "A Collection of Leonardo Da Vinci famous quotes . . . Leonardo Da Vinci, Italian painter, draftsman, sculptor, architect and engineer, 1452–1519." www.thinkexist .com.

2. William Shakespeare, *Measure for Measure,* act 3, scene 1, Duke: Line 35.

3. Thomas Verney and John Kelly, *The Secret Life of the Unborn Child: How You Can Prepare Your Unborn Baby for a Happy, Healthy Life* (New York: Dell, 1981), 73–74.

4. C. Dugovic, S. Maccari, L. Weibel, F. W. Turek, and O. Van Reeth, "Long-Term Effects of Prenatal Stress on Sleep and Circadian Rhythms in Adult Rats," *Sleep Research Online* 2, supplement 1 (1999): 307.

5. Ibid.

6. Thomas Verney and John Kelly, "Some Aspects of Prenatal Parenting," Office of Patient Education, University of Utah Hospitals and Clinics, Document 795, 1999.

7. Ibid.

8. P. G. Hepper, "Fetal Memory: Does It Exist? What Does It Do?" *Acta Paediatrica,* supplement 416 (1996): 16–20.

9. P. G. Hepper, "Fetal 'Soap' Addiction," *Lancet* (June 11, 1988): 1347–48.

10. Ibid.

11. J. W. Goldkrand and B. L. Litvack, "Demonstration of Fetal Habituation and

Patterns of Fetal Heart Response to Vibroacoustic Stimulation in Normal High-Risk Pregnancies," *Obstetrics Gynecology* 24 (1984): 251–56.

12. David Chamberlain, "Prenatal Memory and Learning," Reprinted on Dr. Chamberlain's website: www.birthpsychology.com.

13. Thomas Verney and John Kelly, *The Secret Life of the Unborn Child* (New York: Dell, 1981), 21.

14. Joseph Chilton Pearce, *Magical Child*, 43.

15. Ibid.

16. Ibid.

17. Ibid.

18. J. Atkinson and O. Braddick, "Sensory and Perceptual Capacities of the Prenate," *Psychobiology of the Human Newborn,* ed. Paul Stratton (London: John Wiley, 1982), 191–220.

19. R. Apfelbach, A. Engelhart, P. Bettnisch, and H. Hagenmaierh, "The Olfactory System as a Portal for Airborne Polychlorinated Biphenyls (PCBs) to the Brain," *Archives Toxicology* 72, no. 5 (1998): 314–17.

20. www.riverwatch.com/smell_olfactory_pcb_pcbs.html.

21. Verney and Kelly, *The Secret Life of the Unborn Child,* 45.

22. David Chamberlain, "Babies Remember Pain," *Pre- and Perinatal Psychology Journal* (Summer 1989).

23. Ibid.

24. Ibid.

25. J. Birnholz, J. Stephens, and M. Faria, "Fetal Movement Patterns: A Possible Means of Defining Neurologic Developmental Milestones In Utero," *American Journal of Roentology* 130 (1979): 537–40.

26. David Chamberlain, "Communication before Language," www.birthpsychology.com/lifebefore/comm.html.

27. J. Mannella and G. Beauchamp, "The Transfer of Alcohol to Human Milk: Effects on Flavor and the Infant's Behavior," *New England Journal of Medicine* 325 (1991): 981–85.

28. J. Mannella and G. Beauchamp, "Maternal Diet Alters the Sensory Qualities of Human Milk and the Nursling's Behavior," *Pediatrics* 88 (1991): 737–44.

29. S. Kozuma, A. Nemoto, T. Okai, and M. Minzumo, "Maturational Sequence of Fetal Breathing Movements," *Biology of the Neonate* 60 (1991): 36–40.

30. N. Horimoto, P. Hepper, S. Shahidullah, and T. Koyanagi, "Fetal Eye Movements," *Obstetrics and Gynecology* 3 (1993): 362–69.

31. F. Renggli, "Tracing the Roots of Panic to Prenatal Trauma," in Leonard Schmidt and Brooke Warner, eds., *Panic: Origins, Insight, and Treatment* (Berkeley: North Atlantic Books, 2002).

32. Jeffrey A. Lieberman, "Fetal Growth Restriction Has a Significant Effect on Brain Development and Ultimate Neurodevelopmental Outcome," *Fetal Growth and Development*, cited in *The American Psychiatric Publishing Textbook of Schizophrenia* (2001).

33. G. Spangler, M. Schieche, U. Ilg, U. Maier, and C. Ackerman, "Maternal Sensitivity as an External Organizer for Behavioral Regulation in Infancy," *Developmetal Psychobiology* 7 (1994): 425–37.

34. B. Lipton, "Nature, Nurture, and Human Development," and "The Biology of Conscious Parenting, the New Science of How Parents Shape the Character and Potential of Their Child's Life," January 20, 2008. www.brucelipton .com.

35. Ibid.

36. Barbara Findeisen, review of Dr. Lipton's video, "Nature, Nurture, and the Power of Love: The Biology of Conscious Parenting, the New Science of How Parents Shape the Character and Potential of Their Child's Life," *Journal of Prenatal and Perinatal Psychology and Health* 17, no. 4 (Summer 2003): 335–36.

37. Ibid.

38. Ibid.

39. Ibid.

40. Ibid.

41. Ibid

42. From an article reprinted on Dr. David Chamberlain's website: www .birthpsychology.com.

43. Ibid.

CHAPTER 4. BIRTH: LABOR AND DELIVERY

1. Dick Read, *Childbirth without Fear: The Principles and Practice of Natural Childbirth* (London: Pinter and Martin, Ltd., 2007). Foreword by Michel Odent.

2. Sarah J. Buckley, "Undisturbed Birth: Nature's Blueprint for Ease and Ecstasy," *Journal of Prenatal and Perinatal Psychology and Health* 17, no. 4 (Summer 2003).

3. J. A. Russell, A. J. Douglas, and C. D. Ingram, "The Brain Prepares for Maternity. Adaptive Changes in Behavioral and Neuroendocrine Systems during Pregnancy and Lactation: an Overview," *Prog Brain Res* 133:1–38 [Medline], 2001.

4. Jackson and Dudley, "Estrogen Increases Oxytocin Receptor Sites after Full Cervical Dilatation," *Journal of Clinical Endocrinology & Metabolism,* June 1998.

5. Verbalis, McCann, McHale, and Strickler, *Investing in Women,* A publication of a group of the same name that built strong ties with women's groups and local business. "The Mention of the Oxytocin Effect," 1998.

6. Michel Odent, "The Fetal Ejection Reflex," *The Nature of Birth and Breastfeeding* (Westport, Conn.: Bergin and Garvey, 1992).

7. Buckley, "Undisturbed Birth: Nature's Blueprint for Ease and Ecstasy."

8. R. S. Goland, S. L. Wardlow, M. Blum, P. J. Tropper, and R. I. Stark, "Biologically Active Corticotrophin-Releasing Hormone in Maternal and Fetal Plasma during Pregnancy," *American Journal of Obstetrics and Gynecology* 159 (1989): 884–90.

9. C. Kimball, "Do Endorphin Residues of Beta Lipotrophin in Hormone Reinforce Reproductive Functions?" *American Journal of Obstetrics and Gynecology* 134, no. 2 (1979): 127–32.

10. L. Irestedt, H. Lagercrantz and P. Belfrage, "Causes and Consequences of Maternal and Fetal Sympathoadrenal Activation during Parturition," *Acta Obstretrica Gynecologica Scandinavica,* supplement 1, no. 18 (1984): 111–15.

11. D. R. Grattan, "The Actions of Prolactin in the Brain during Pregnancy and Lactation," *Progress in Brain Research* 135 (2001): 153–71.

12. R. E. Gilbert and P. A. Tookey, "Perinatal Mortality and Morbidity among Babies Delivered in Water: National Surveillance Study," *British Medical Journal* 319 (1999): 483–87.

13. Hafner-Eaton and Pearce, *Journal of Health Policies,* Policy and Law 19, no. 4 (1994): 813–35.

14. H. C. Woodcock, W. W. Read, C. Bower, C. Stanley, and F. J. Moore, *Midwifery* 10, no. 3 (September 1994): 125–35.

15. S. Cherniske, *The DHEA Breakthrough* (New York: Balantine, 1998); J. Hopper, "Ommm . . . Please Pass the DHEA," *Health Magazine* 21 (1989): 34; Kabat-Zinn, *Full Catastrophe Living: Using the Wisdom of Your Body and Mind to Face Stress, Pain, and Illness* (New York: Bantam Doubleday Dell,

1990); C. Pert, *Molecules of Emotion* (New York: Simon and Schuster, 1997); W. Pierpaoli and W. Regelson, *The Melatonin Miracle* (New York: Simon and Schuster, 1995).

16. Robert Newman, "Sharing Space: Childbirth Meditation and Advanced Natural Childbirth," *Journal of Prenatal and Perinatal Psychology and Health* 17, no. 4 (Summer 2003): 321–31.

17. H. Benson, *Timeless Healing: The Power and Biology of Belief* (New York: Simon and Schuster, 1993).

18. Newman, "Sharing Space: Childbirth Meditation and Advanced Natural Childbirth," 331.

19. Nancy Griffin, "Let the Baby Decide," *Mothering Magazine* (March/April, 2001): 69.

20. Christiane Northrup, *Women's Bodies, Women's Wisdom* (New York: Bantam, 1998).

21. David Stewart, *The Five Standards of Safe Childbearing* (National Association of Parents & Professionals for Safe Alternative Childbirth [NAPSAC], 1998), revised ed.

22. G. Bacigalupo, S. Riese, H. Rosendahl, and E. Saling, "Quantitative Relationships between Pain Intensities during Labor and Beta-Endorphin and Cortisol Concentrations in Plasma: Decline of the Hormone Concentrations in the Early Postpartum," *Journal of Perinatal Medicine* 18, no. 4 (1990): 289–96.

23. D. Krehbiel, P. Poindron, F. Levy, and M. J. Prud'Homme, "Peridural Anesthesia Disturbs Maternal Behavior in Primiparous and Multiparous Parturient Ewes," *Physiology and Behavior* 40 (1987): 463–72.

24. C. B. Sepkoski, G. Lester, G. W. Ostheimer, and B. Brazelton, "The Effects of Maternal Epidural Anesthesia on Neonatal Behavior during the First Month," *Developmental Medicine and Child Neurology* 34 (1992): 1072–80.

25. J. Riordan, A. S. Gross, J. Angeron, B. Krumwiede, and J. Melin, "The Effect of Labor Pain Relief Medication on Neonatal Suckling and Breast-Feeding Duration," *Journal of Human Lactation* 16, no. 1 (2000): 7–12.

26. D. J. Baumgarten, P. Muehl, M. Fischer, and B. Pribbenow, "Effect of Labor Epidural Anesthesia on Breast Feeding of Healthy Full-Term Newborns Delivered Vaginally," *Journal of American Board of Family Practice* 16, no. 1 (2003): 7–13.

27. Linda J. Mayberry, Donna Clemmens, and Anindya De, "Epidural Anealgesia Side Effects, Interventions and Care of Women during Childbirth: A System-

atic Review," *American Journal of Obstetrics and Gynecology* 186, issue 5 (May 2002): S81–S93.

28. D. A. Luthy, K. K. Shy, et al., "Effects of Electronic Fetal Heart Rate Monitoring," *New England Journal of Medicine* (March 1, 1990): 588–93.

29. Janet Tipton, ed., *Is Homebirth for You: Six Myths About Childbirth Exposed* (Big Sandy, Tex.: Friends of Homebirth, 1990).

30. Milton Singer, *The Cutting Edge,* (New York: E. P. Dutton, 1990).

31. K. A. Bidgood and P. J. Steer, "A Randomized Control Study of Oxytocin Augmentation of Labor: 2. Uterine Activity," *British Journal of Obstetrics and Gynecology* 94, no. 6 (1987): 518–22.

32. L. Gilbert, W. Porter, and V. Brown, "Postpartum Hemorrhage: A Continuing Problem," *British Journal of Obstetrics and Gynecology* 94 (1987): 67–71.

33. E. A. Friedman and M. R. Sachtleben, "Affect of Oxytocin and Oral Prostaglandin E2 on Uterine Contractility and Fetal Heart Rate Patterns," *American Journal of Obstetrics and Gynecology* 130, no. 4 (1978): 403–7.

34. Michel Odent, "The Fetus Ejection Reflex," in *The Nature of Birth and Breast Feeding* (Westport, Conn.: Bergin and Garvey, 1992).

35. Ibid.

36. P. Shiono, et. al., "Mid-Line Episiotomies: More Harm than Good?" *American Journal of Obstetrics and Gynecology* (May 1990): 765–70.

37. Christiane Northrup, *Women's Bodies, Women's Wisdom: Creating Physical and Emotional Health and Healing* (New York: Bantam, 1998).

38. G. Faxelius, K. Hagnevik, H. Lagercrantz, B. Lundell, and I. Irestedt, "Catecholamine Surge and Lung Function after Delivery," *Archives of Disease in Childhood* 58, no. 4 (1983): 262–66.

39. E. Hemminki and J. Merilainen, "Long-Term Effects of Cesarean Section: Ectopic Pregnancies and Placental Problems," *American Journal of Obstetrics and Gynecology* 174, no. 5 (1996): 1569–74.

40. Nancy Cohen and Louis J. Estner, *Silent Knife: Cesarian Prevention and Vaginal Birth after Cesarian* (Westport, Conn.: Bergin and Garvey, 1983).

41. J. Fischer, J. Astbury, and A. Smith, "Adverse Psychological Impact of Operative Obstetric Interventions: A Prospective Longitudinal Study," *Australia New Zealand Journal of Psychiatry* 31 (1997): 728–38.

42. Pearce, *Magical Child.*

43. Erasmus Darwin, *Zoonomia or the Laws of Organic Life* vol. 3 (London: n.p., 1801), 321.

44. G. M. Morley, "Cord Closure: Does Hasty Clamping Injure the Newborn?" *Obgyn Management* (July 1998): 29–36.

45. www.cordclamping.com/History.htm.

46. T. Peltonen, "Placental Transfusion, Advantage-Disadvantage," *European Journal of Pediatrics* 137 (1981): 141–46.

47. O. Linderkamp, "Placental Transfusion: Determinants and Effects," *Clinics in Perinatology* 9 (1982): 559–92.

48. S. Kinmond, et. al., "Umbilical Cord Clamping and Preterm Infants: A Randomized Trail," *British Medical Journal* 306 (1993): 172–75.

49. S. Buckley, "Don't Clamp the Cord," article at www.lotusbirth.com.

50. R. Usher, M. Shepherd, and J. Lind, "The Blood Volume of the Newborn Infant and Placental Transfusion," *Acta Paediatrica Scandanavica* 52 (1963): 497–512.

51. G. M. Morley, "How the Cord Clamp Injures Your Baby's Brain," 2004, available on www.whale.to/a/cord.html and www.cordclamping.com.

52. Ibid.

53. Ibid.

54. Ibid.

CHAPTER 5. BREASTFEEDING

1. Dr. William Sears, *The Baby Book* (Boston: Little Brown, 1992).

2. The World Health Organization's infant feeding recommendation-WHA54 A54/ INF.DOC./4 - Global strategy for infant and young child feeding. The optimal duration of exclusive breastfeeding Provisional agenda item 13.1, 1 May 2001.

3. Ibid.

4. Dr. Miriam Labbok, "Breastfeeding: The Best Choice for Babies," UNICEF Nutrition, August 1, 2005.

5. David Meyers, "Promoting and Supporting Breastfeeding," *American Family Physician* (September 15, 2001).

6. L. John Horwood and David M. Fergusson, "Breastfeeding and Later Cognitive and Academic Outcomes," *Pediatrics* 101, no. 1 (January 1998): 9.

7. Ibid., 91–97.

8. M. Niculescu, S. Zeisel, and Y. Yamamuro, "Breastfeeding Increases Choline, Which Means More Brain Cells," *Journal of Neurochem* (April 2004).

9. Much of the information in this section is featured on the website, www.AskDrSears.com, the section on breastfeeding.

10. A. Singhai, "Breast Milk May Prevent Later Heart Disease," *Lancet* (May 14, 2004).

11. J. Koenig, A. Davies, and B. Thach, "Coordination of Breathing, Sucking and Swallowing during Bottle Feedings in Human Infants," *Journal of Applied Physiology* 69 (1990): 1623–29.

12. Joseph Chilton Pearce, *Magical Child Matures* (New York: Dutton, 1985), 30.

13. American Academy of Pediatrics, "Work Group of Breastfeeding," *Pediatrics* 100 (1997): 1035–39.

14. Reported on Dr. William Sears' website, www.AskDrSears.com. See the section on breastfeeding.

15. Ibid.

16. "Protein in Human Milk Reduces Risk of Obesity," posted by News-Medical. Net in *Medical Study News* (May 3, 2004) and reported on www.News-Medical.net.

17. Reported on Dr. William Sears' website, www.AskDrSears.com. See the section on breastfeeding.

18. P. R. Erickson and E. Mazhare, "Investigation of the Role of Human Breast Milk in Caries Development," *Pediatrics Dentistry* 21 (1999): 86–90.

19. "Breastfeeding Can Reduce the Risk of Death for Infants in Their First Year of Life," posted by News-Medical.Net in *Child Health News* (May 3, 2004) and reported on www.News-Medical.net.

20. A. Harvieux, M. McClain, P. Tackitt, K. Fernbach, R. McCoy, and C. Hunt, *Breastfeeding, Sudden Infant Death Syndrome, and a Safe Sleep Environment* (Stony Brook, N.Y.: Association of SIDS and Infant Mortality Programs, New York State Center for SIDS, School of Social Welfare, 2001).

21. M. Bosco, *Breastfeeding and Reduction of SIDS* (North Andover, Mass.: Fitzgerald Health Education Associates, 2004).

22. www.breastfeeding.com.

23. Ibid.

24. Ibid.

25. Ibid.

26. Ibid.

27. Ibid.

28. Ibid.

29. Ibid.

30. Ibid.

31. Ibid.

32. Ibid.

33. Ibid.

34. Ibid.

35. Ibid.

36. Ibid.

37. Ibid.

38. A. Dermer, "A Well-Kept Secret: Breastfeeding's Benefits to Mothers," *New Beginnings* 18, no.4 (July–August, 2001).

39. A. P. Schneider, "Risk Factor for Ovarian Cancer," *New England Journal of Medicine* (1987).

40. www.cancer.org.

41. K. E. Brock, "Sexual, Reproductive, and Contraceptive Risk Factors for Carcinoma-in-situ of the Uterine Cervix in Sidney," *Medical Journal of Australia* (1989).

42. "Breastfeeding and Fertility," reported on Dr. William Sears' website, www .AskDrSears.com. See the section on breastfeeding.

43. C. Jorgensen, et. al., "Oral Contraception, Parity, Breastfeeding, and Severity of Rheumatoid Arthritis," *Annual Rheumatic Dis* 5 (1996): 94.

44. La Leche League at www.llli.org to learn more about La Leche League International and mothering through breastfeeding.

45. A. Dermer, "A Well-Kept Secret: Breastfeeding's Benefits to Mothers," *New Beginnings* 18, no.4 (July–August, 2001).

46. Sears, *The Baby Book.*

CHAPTER 6. LIFE AFTER BIRTH:
THE MOST IMPORTANT DAYS OF OUR LIVES

1. Carlos Castaneda, *Tales of Power* (New York: Simon and Schuster, 1975).

2. Pearce, *Magical Child Matures,* 27.

3. Michel Odent, *The Scientification of Love* (London: Free Association Books, 2001), 2.

4. J. Terkel and J. S. Rosenblatt, "Maternal Behavior Induced by Maternal Blood Plasma Injected into Virgin Rats," *Journal of Comparative Physiological Psychology* 65 (1968): 479–82.

5. Odent, *The Scientification of Love,* 12.

6. A. Raine, P. Brennan, and S. A. Medink, "Birth Complications Combined

with Early Maternal Rejection at Age 1 Year Predispose to Violent Crime at 18 Years," *Archives of General Psychiatry* 51 (1994): 984–88.

7. R. Hattori, et al., "Autistic Developmental Disorders after General Anesthesia Delivery," 337 *Lancet* (June 1, 1991): 1357–58.

8. N. Tinbergen and Elizabeth A. Tinbergen, *Autistic Children: New Hope for a Cure* (London: Allen and Unwin, 1983).

9. Odent, *The Scientification of Love,* 18.

10. H. Forssman and J. Thuwe, "Continued Follow-Up Study of 120 Persons Born after Refusal of Application for Therapeutic Abortion," *Acta Psychiatrics Scandinavica* 64 (1981): 142–49.

11. Pearce, *Magical Child Matures,* 28.

12. Ibid.

13. C. Sherrington, *Man on His Nature* (London: Penguin, 1995), 147.

14. G. Doherty-Sneddon, *Children's Unspoken Language* (London: Jessica Kingsley Publishers, 2003).

15. Pearce, *Magical Child,* 53.

16. William Sears, "Bonding with Your Newborn," *Attachment Parenting International Journal,* www.attachmentparenting.org.

17. N. Bergman, "Kangaroo Mother Care," video (Geddes Productions, 2001). Visit www.geddespro.com to order this highly informative video.

18. Pearce, *Magical Child Matures.*

19. R. Ferber, *Solve Your Child's Sleep Problems* (New York: Simon and Schuster, 1985).

20. W. Caudil and H. Weinstein, "Maternal Care and Infant Behavior in Japan and America," *Psychiatry* 32 (1969): 12–43.

21. T. Barry Brazelton, "Parent-Infant Co-Sleeping Revisited," *Ab Initio* 2, no. 1 (1990).

22. G. A. Morelli, et al., "Cultural Variation in Infant's Sleeping Arrangements: Questions of Independence," *Developmental Psychology* 28 (1992): 604–13.

23. P. Heron, "Nonreactive Co-Sleeping and Child Behavior. Getting a Good Night's Sleep All Night Every Night," masters thesis, University of Bristol, England, 1964.

24. J. F. Forbes, D. S. Weiss, and R. A. Folen, "The Co-Sleeping Habits of Military Children," *Military Medicine* 15, no. 7 (1992): 196–200.

25. J. Mosenkis, "The Effects of Childhood Co-Sleeping on Later Life Development," masters thesis, University of Chicago, 1998.

26. W. G. Guntheroth and P. Spiers, "Sleeping Prone and the Risk of the Sudden Infant Death Syndrome," *Journal of American Medical Association* 2 (1992): 359–63.

27. J. McKenna, "Cultural Influences on Infant Sleep," in J. Loughlin, J. Carroll, and C. Marcus, eds., *Sleep and Breathing in Children: A Developmental Approach* (New York: Marcel Dekker, 2000).

28. Ibid.

29. S. Mosko, et al., "Mutual Behavioral and Psychological Influences among Solitary and Co-Sleeping Mother-Infant Pairs," *Early Human Development* 38 (1994): 182–201.

30. M. N. Ozturk and O. M. Ozturk, "Thumbsucking and Falling Asleep," *British Journal of Medical Psychology* 50 (1977): 95–103.

31. M. F. Elias, "Sleep-Wake Patterns of Breast-Fed Infants in the First Two Years of Life," *Pediatrics* 77, no. 3 (1986): 322–29.

32. J. McKenna, "Cultural Influences on Infant Sleep," in J. Loughlin, J. Carroll, and C. Marcus, eds., *Sleep and Breathing in Children: A Developmental Approach* (New York: Marcel Dekker, 2000).

CHAPTER 7. THE GREAT HEALER

1. Robbie Davis-Floyd and Elizabeth Davis, "Intuition as Authoritative Knowledge in Midwifery and Home Birth," in *Childbirth and Authoritative Knowledge,* edited by Robbie Davis-Floyd and Carolyn Sargent (Los Angeles: University of California Press, 1997), 316.

2. Jean Liedoff, cited in Joseph Chilton Pearce, *Magical Parent Magical Child* (Nevada City, Calif.: In-Joy Publications, 2002), 22.

3. Ibid.

4. Joseph Chilton Pearce, "The Conflict of Interest between Biological and Cultural Imperatives," *Touch The Future* (Spring 2004): 8.

5. Pearce, *Magical Parent Magical Child,* 55.

Bibliography

Acuff, Daniel S., and Robert H. Reiher. *Kidnapped: How Irresponsible Marketers Are Stealing the Minds of Your Children.* Chicago: Dearborn, 2005.

Ainsworth, Mary, M.D. "Deprivation of Maternal Care: A Reassessment of Its Effect," *Public Health Papers,* no. 14, pp. 97–165. Geneva: World Health Organization, n.d.

———. *Immaculate Deception: A New Look at Women and Childbirth in America.* Boston: Houghton Mifflin, 1975.

———. *Infancy in Uganda.* Baltimore: Johns Hopkins University Press, 1967.

Albert, David. *And the Skylark Sings With Me: Adventures in Homeschooling and Community-Based Education.* Gabriola Island, British Columbia: New Society Publishers, 1999.

———. *Have Fun, Learn Stuff, Grow: Homeschooling and the Curriculum of Love.* Monroe, Maine: Common Courage Press, 2006.

———. *The Healing Heart-Families: Storytelling to Encourage Caring and Healthy Families.* Gabriola Island, British Columbia: New Society Publishers, 2003.

———. *Homeschooling and the Voyage of Self Discovery: A Journey of Original Seeking.* Monroe, Maine: Common Courage Press, 2003.

———. *The Healing Heart-Communities: Storytelling to Build Strong and Healthy Communities.* Gabriola Island, British Columbia: New Society Publishers, 2003.

Albert, David, and Joyce Reed. "What Really Matters." *Natural Life Magazine,* 2009.

Arms, Suzanne. *Immaculate Deception: A New Look at Women and Childbirth in America.* Boston: Houghton Mifflin Company, 1975.

Bartalanfy, Ludwig Von. *A Systems View of Man.* Edited by Paul LaViolette. Boulder, Colo.: Westview Press 1981.

Bateson, Gregory. *Mind and Nature: A Necessary Unity*. New York: E. P. Dutton, 1979.

Berends, Polly Berrien. *Whole Child/Whole Parent*. New York: Harper and Row, 1988.

Bernard, J., and L. Sontag. "Fetal Reactions to Sound." *Journal of Genetic Psychology* no. 70 (1947): 209–10.

Blake, William. *Selected Poetry and Prose*. New York: The Modern Library, Random House, 1953.

Bohm, David. *Causality and Chance in Modern Physics*. Philadelphia: University of Pennsylvania Press, 1971.

———. "Insight Knowledge, Science and Human Values." *Education and Values*. Edited by Douglas Sloan. New York: Teachers College Press, Columbia University, 1980.

———. *Wholeness and the Implicate Order*. London: Routledge and Kegan Paul, 1979.

Bolby, John. "The Child's Tie to His Mother: Attachment Behavior." *Attachment and Loss* 1. New York: Basic Books, 1969, 1980.

Brackbill, Yvonne. "Effects of Obstetric Drugs on Human Development." Presented at the conference: Obstetrical Management and Infant Outcome, American Foundation for Maternal and Child Health, November 1979.

Bradshaw, John. *Bradshaw on the Family: A Revolutionary Way of Self Discovery*. Deerfield Beach, Fla.: Health Communications, Inc., 1988.

Buckley, Sarah. "Undisturbed Birth: Nature's Blueprint for Ease and Ecstasy." *Journal of Prenatal and Perinatal Psychology and Health* 17, no. 4 (Summer 2003): 261–89.

Buhner, Stephen Harrod. *The Secret Teachings of Plants: The Intelligence of the Heart in the Direct Perception of Nature*. Rochester, Vt.: Bear and Co., 2004.

Caplan, Mariana. *Untouched: The Need for Genuine Affection in an Impersonal World*. Prescott, Ariz.: Hohm Press, 1998.

Carlebach, Shlomo, with Susan Yael Mesinai. *Shlomo's Stories, Selected Tales*. Northvale, N.J.: Jason Aronson, 1997.

Carroll, David. *Spiritual Parenting*. New York: Marlowe, 1990.

Castaneda, Carlos. *Tales of Power*. New York: Simon and Schuster, 1976.

———. *The Teachings of Don Juan*. New York: Simon and Schuster, 1970.

Chamberlain, David. *Babies Remember Birth*. Los Angeles: Jeremy P. Tarcher, 1988.

———. *Consciousness at Birth: A Review of the Empirical Evidence.* San Diego: Chamberlain Publications, 2000.

Condon, W., and Louis Sander. "Neonate Movement Is Synchronized with Adult Speech: Interactional Participation and Language Acquisition." *Science* (January 1974).

Davis-Floyd, Robbie. *Birth as an American Rite of Passage.* Berkeley: University of California Press, 1992.

———. *Birth in Four Cultures: A Cross-cultural Investigation of Childbirth in Yucatan, Holland, Sweden, and the United States.* Brigitte Jordan. Revised and expanded by Robbie Davis-Floyd. Prospect Heights, Ill.: Waveland Press, Inc. 1993.

Davis-Floyd, Robbie, and Joseph Dumit. *Cyborg Babies: From Techno-Sex to Techno-Tots.* New York: Routledge, 1998.

Davis-Floyd, Robbie, and Carolyn Sargent. "The Anthropology of Birth." *Childbirth and Authoritative Knowledge.* Berkeley and Los Angeles: University of California Press, 1997.

Dossey, Larry, M.D. *Space, Time, and Medicine.* Boulder, Colo.: Shambhala, 1982.

Eberstadt, Mary. *Home Alone in America: The Hidden Toll of Day Care, Behavioral Drugs, and Other Parent Substitutes.* New York: Sentinel, 2004.

Fodor, J. A. "Speech Discrimination in Infants." *Perception and Psychophysics* 18, no. 2 (1975).

French, R. M., trans. *The Way of a Pilgrim.* New York: Seabury Press, 1965.

Gaskin, Ina May. *Spiritual Midwifery.* New York: Schocken, 1975.

Gatto, John Taylor. *Dumbing Us Down: The Hidden Curriculum of Compulsory Schooling.* Gabriola Island, British Columbia: New Society Publishers, 1992.

Geber, Marcelle. "The Psycho-Motor Development of African Children in the First Year and the Influence of Maternal Behavior." *Journal of Social Psychology,* no. 37 (1958).

Glas, Norbert. *Conception, Birth and Early Childhood.* Spring Valley, N.Y.: Anthroposophic Press (1972).

Grey, Alex. *The Sacred Mirrors.* Rochester, Vt.: Inner Traditions, 1990.

———. *Transfigurations.* Rochester, Vt.: Inner Traditions, 2001.

Grof, Stanislav, M.D. *Realms of the Human Unconscious.* New York: E. P. Dutton, 1976.

Gurdjieff, George I. *Views from the Real World.* New York: E. P. Dutton, 1975.

Harlow, Harry F. "Love in Infant Monkeys." *Scientific American* (June 1959).

Harlow, Harry F., and Margaret Harlow. "Social Deprivation in Monkeys." *Scientific American* (1962).

Hartmann, Thom. *The Last Hours of Ancient Sunlight: the Fate of the World and What We Can Do Before It's Too Late.* New York: Three Rivers Press, 2004.

———. *The Prophet's Way: A Guide to Living in the Now.* Rochester, Vt.: Park Street Press, 2004.

Holt, John. *How Children Learn.* Series: Classics in Child Development. Cambridge, Mass.: Perseus Books, 1995.

———. *Instead of Education: Ways to Help People Do Things Better.* New York: E. P. Dutton, 1976.

Hughes, Laurel. *How to Raise Good Children: Encouraging Moral Growth.* Nashville: Abingdon Press, 1988.

Hunt, Jan. *The Natural Child, Parenting from the Heart.* Gabriola Island, British Columbia: New Society Publishers, 2001.

Illich, Ivan. *Medical Nemesis.* New York: Pantheon Books, 1976.

Jackson, Deborah. *Three in a Bed: Why You Should Sleep with Your Baby.* London: Bloomsbury, 1989.

Jordan, Brigitte. "Authoritive Knowledge." *Childbirth and Authoritative Knowledge.* Berkeley and Los Angeles: University of California Press, 1997.

Kennell, John, H., and Marshall H. Klaus. "Early Mother-Infant Contact: Effects on Breastfeeding." *Breastfeeding and Food Policy in a Hungry World.* New York: Academic Press, 1979.

Khan, Hazrat Inayat. *The Sufi Message.* Volume 3. London: Barrie and Jenkins, 1971.

Klaus, Marshall. "Maternal Attachment: Importance of the First Post-Partum Days." *New England Journal of Medicine,* no. 9 (1972).

Konig, Karl. *The First Three Years of the Child.* New York: Anthroposophic Press, 1969.

Leach, Penelope. *Children First: What Our Society Must Do—and Is Not Doing—for Our Children.* New York: Alfred A. Knopf, 1994.

LeBoyer, Frederick. *Birth without Violence.* New York: Knopf, 1974.

Lehman, Christine. "Young Brains Don't Distinguish Real from Televised Violence." *Psychiatric News* 39, no. 15 (2004).

Liedloff, Jean. *The Continuum Concept: In Search of Happiness Lost.* Cambridge, Mass.: Perseus Books, 1985.

Lipton, Bruce. *The Biology of Belief: Unleashing the Power of Consciousness, Matter, and Miracles.* Santa Rosa, Calif.: Mountain of Love/Elite Books, 2005.

MacLean, Paul. *A Triune Concept of the Brain and Behavior.* Clarence M. Hines Memorial Lecture Series. Edited by D. Campbell and T. J. Boag. Toronto: University of Toronto Press, 1973.

———. *The Triune Brain in Evolution: Role in Palerocerebral Functions.* New York: Plenum Press, 1990.

Mandelbaum, Yitta Halberstam. *Holy Brother: Inspiring Stories and Enchanted Tales about Rabbi Shlomo Carlebach.* Northvale, N.J.: Jason Aronson, 1997.

Mander, Jerry. *Four Arguments for the Elimination of Television.* New York: Perennial Books, 2002.

Mendizza, Michael, and Joseph Chilton Pearce. *Magical Parent Magical Child: The Optimum Learning Relationship.* Nevada City: In-Joy Publications, 2002.

Miller, Alice. *For Your Own Good: Hidden Cruelty in Child-Rearing and the Roots of Violence.* New York: The Noon Day Press, 1990.

———. *Thou Shalt Not Be Aware: Society's Betrayal of the Child.* New York: Meridian, New American Library, 1986.

Montagu, Ashley. *Life Before Birth.* New York: New American Library, 1964.

———. *The Natural Superiority of Women.* New York: Macmillan, 1968.

———. *Touching: The Human Significance of Skin.* New York: Columbia University Press, 1971.

Neil, A. S. *Summerhill School: A New View of Childhood.* New York: St. Martin's Griffon, 1995.

Northrup, Christiane. *Women's Bodies, Women's Wisdom: Creating Physical and Emotional Health and Healing.* New York: Bantam Books, 1998.

Odent, Michel. *The Caesarean.* London: Free Association Books, 2004.

———. *The Scientification of Love.* London: Free Association Books, 2001.

Ornstein, Robert. *The Nature of Human Consciousness (A Book of Readings).* New York: Viking Press, 1973.

———. *The Psychology of Consciousness.* San Francisco: Miller Freeman Publications, 1971.

Ouspensky, P. D. *In Search of the Miraculous: Fragments of an Unknown Teaching.* New York: Harcourt, Brace and World, Inc., 1949.

———. *The Psychology of Man's Possible Evolution.* New York: Hedgehog Press Inc., 1950.

Pearce, Joseph Chilton. *The Biology of Transcendence: A Blueprint of the Human Spirit.* Rochester, Vt.: Park Street Press, 2002.

———. *Bond of Power: Meditation and Prayer.* New York: Dutton, 1981.

———. *The Crack in the Cosmic Egg: New Constructs of Mind and Reality.* Rochester, Vt.: Park Street Press, 2002.

———. *Magical Child.* New York: Dutton, 1977.

———. *Magical Child Matures.* New York: Dutton, 1985.

Piaget, Jean. *The Child's Conception of the World.* New York: Humanities Press, 1951.

———. *The Origins of Intelligence in Children.* New York: International University Press, 1952.

———. *Play, Dreams, and Imitation in Children.* New York: W. W. Norton, 1962.

Piaget, Jean, and B. Inhelder. *The Early Growth of Logic in the Child.* Atlantic Highlands, N.J.: Humanities Press, 1964.

Penfield, Wilder. *The Mystery of the Mind: A Critical Study of Consciousness and the Human Brain.* Princeton, N.J.: Princeton University Press, 1975.

Prescott, James. "The Origins of Human Love and Violence." Institute of Humanistic Science Monograph, 7th International Congress, Association for Pre- and Perinatal Psychology and Health, 1997.

Raphael, Dana. *The Tender Gift of Breastfeeding.* New York: Schocken Books, 1978.

Renggli, Franz. "Tracing the Roots of Panic to Prenatal Trauma." *Journal of Prenatal and Perinatal Psychology and Health* 17, no. 4 (Summer 2003): 289–301.

Rhoades, Steven. *Taking Sex Differences Seriously.* San Francisco: Encounter Books, 2004.

Rosenberg, Marshall B. *Nonviolent Communication: A Language of Compassion.* Del Mar, Calif.: PuddleDancer Press, 1999.

Roszak, Theodore. *Ecopsychology: Restoring the Earth, Healing the Mind.* San Francisco, Calif.: Sierra Club Books, 1995.

Sears, Martha. *The Breastfeeding Book: Everything You Need to Know about Nursing Your Child from Birth through Weaning.* Boston: Little Brown, 2000.

Sears, Martha, and William Sears. *The Attachment Parenting Book: A Common Sense Guide to Understanding and Nurturing Your Baby.* Boston: Little Brown, 2002.

———. *The Baby Book: Everything You Need to Know about Your Baby from Birth to Age Two.* Boston: Little Brown, 2003.

Sheldrake, Rupert. *A New Science of Life: The Hypothesis of Formative Causation.* Rochester, Vt.: Park Street Press, 1995.

———. *Dogs That Know When Their Masters Are Coming Home and Other Unexplained Powers of Animals.* New York: Three Rivers Press, 1999.

———. *The Sense of Being Stared At: And Other Unexplained Powers of the Mind.* New York: Crown, 2003.

Shore, Allan. *Affect Regulation and the Origin of Self.* Hillsdale, N.J.: Lawrence Erlbaum Associates, 1994.

Small, Meredith F. *Kids: How Biology and Culture Shape the Way We Raise Children.* New York: Doubleday, 2001.

———. *Our Babies, Our Selves: How Biology and Culture Shape the Way We Parent.* New York: Anchor Books, 1998.

Speeth, Kathleen Riordan. *The Gurdjieff Work.* Berkeley, Calif.: And/Or Press, 1976.

Storfer, Miles. *Intelligence and Giftedness: The Contributions of Heredity and Early Environment.* San Francisco: Jossey-Bass, 1989.

Thevenin, Tine. *The Family Bed: An Age-Old Concept in Child Rearing.* P.O. Box 16004, Minneapolis, Minnesota 55416, 1976.

Velmans, William, *Understanding Consciousness.* London: Routledge, 2000.

Verney, Thomas, and John Kelly. *The Secret Life of the Unborn Child: How You Can Prepare Your Unborn Child for a Happy and Healthy Life.* New York: Dell, 1981.

Welch, Martha. *Holding Time.* New York: Fireside, 1988.

Windle, W. F. "Brain Damage by Asphyxia." *Scientific American* (October 1969).

Zipf, George Kingsley. *Human Behavior and the Principle of Least Resistance: An Introduction to Human Ecology.* Reading, Mass.: Addison-Wesley Publishers, 1949.

Resources

VIDEOS OF INTEREST

We have chosen these videos for readers who have never seen a birth, let alone a natural birth. They were chosen for their modesty and beauty. There are no scenes that will shock.

Birth

Giving Birth: Challenges and Choices with Suzanne Arms
and Dr. Christiane Northrup
Available from: Birthing The Future, P.O. Box 830, Durango, Co. 81302,
1-877-BIRTHING

Life Before Birth: The Shaping Nature of our Prenatal Experience
Available from: www.quantumparenting.com

The Timeless Way: A History of Birth from Ancient to Modern Times
Available at: In-Joy Videos, 3970 Broadway, Suite B4, Boulder, Co. 80304
1-800-326-2082

www.metacafe.com/watch/yt-gM-A8OZyz7U/isabellas_water_birth_video
Lovely video with the father cutting the umbilical cord. Mostly black-and-white stills with music background.

www.metacafe.com/watch/yt-52-mWneflhY/the_water_birth_of_amazing_grace
Joyous birth with husband and other family members.

www.metacafe.com/watch/yt-7E-wULAaD50/natural_childbirth_of_twins_and_triplets

Amazing testimonials from mothers who naturally birthed twins at home.

www.metacafe.com/watch/yt-r_77qzUY6IQ/live_natural_water_birth_baby_girl

Baby literally popping out in this very short and emotional video.

www.sarahjbuckley.com/html/gentle-birth-gentle-mothering-interview01.htm

An interview with Dr. Sarah Buckley about her book *Gentle Birth, Gentle Mothering* and her insights on epidurals, hormones, and how to have a natural birth.

Breastfeeding

www.5min.com/Video/How-to-Breastfeed-29160917

Simple instructional video.

www.breastfeeding.com

This website offers extensive information and videos on breastfeeding.

Parenting

Babies Know More Than You Think: Exploring the capacity of consciousness of new human beings with David Chamberlain and Suzanne Arms

Available from: Touch the Future, P.O. Box 1447, Ojai, Calif. 93024; or call 805-646-4681; or e-mail: michael@TTFuture.org.

Reveals the scientific evidence for earliest conscious intelligence in newborns.

Holding Time with Dr. Martha Welch

Available from: Dr. Martha Welch, 127 East 59th Street, New York, N.Y. 10022

This original work with difficult, angry, or depressed children shows how physically holding your child for a time alters the behavior in the child. It creates a nonverbal physical bond. Conversation can then be effective in talking to the child.

Nature, Nurture and the Power of Love with Dr. Bruce Lipton

Available from www.holisticpage.com.au/_Bruce_Lipton.php

Dr. Lipton's new discoveries in genetics prove how our genes are not static, as we thought, but change depending on nurture or the lack of it from outside.

The Origins of Love and Violence by Dr. James W. Prescott

Available from: Dr. James W. Prescott, 1140-17 Savannah Road Lewes, DE 19958

jprescott34@comcast.net

This video is a classic. His work with monkeys is very enchanting and proves how nurture brings baby monkeys to the soft artificial mother monkey all day. They only go to the food-providing wire mother for short bursts to eat and return to the cuddly mother.

Joseph Chilton Pearce Video Series

Magical Child

Awakening of Intelligence

Pregnancy, Birth & Bonding

Imagination & Play

Learning and Education

Critical & Creative Thinking

Beyond Adolescence

Available from Touch the Future, P.O. Box 1447, Ojai, Calif. 93024; e-mail: michael@TTFuture.org; call 805-646-4681

This is an unbelievable chance to see and hear the master in this field.

WEBSITES OF INTEREST

Birth

www.askdrsears.com

Dr. Sears answers any question you may have about the day-to-day requirements of attachment parenting.

www.birthintobeing.com

Excellent birthing site that recognizes the important role conscious birth and parenting play in mankind's survival and future.

www.birthpsychology.com/index.html

The website of The Association for Prenatal and Perinatal Psychology and Health. The latest journal articles on prebirth, in utero and birth.

www.birthworks.org/site/primal-health-research.html

Dr. Michel Odent explores the end of the Primal period when we are in a basic state of health called primal health. The objective of primal health research is to explore correlations between the Primal period and what will happen later on.

www.calmbirth.org

A system during pregnancy using progressive/relaxation techniques, moving attention through the whole body to heal the mother's and infant's nervous system of any prenatal disturbances. It offers another form of prenatal bonding.

www.dona.org

Locator for doulas internationally.

home.comcast.net/~cnmpat/pregandmw.html

Pregnancy and midwifery information.

www.icea.org

International Childbirth Education Association

www.midwifeinfo.com

One of the best midwifery sites with the latest news and articles of interest from around the world.

thenewparenting.com

Jeffrey Fine's website contains his Blog and other offerings from the Fines including: online interactive counseling, audio sets on various subjects, podcasts, and upcoming teleseminars.

www.ttfuture.org

Michael Mendizza, author, educator, filmmaker, and founder of Touch the Future Learning Design Center, has a wealth of information for all of us. Reviews and excerpts from leaders in this field are only one example of what is offered on this website.

www.waterbirth.org

All you want to know about this interesting alternative of water birth.

www.wombecology.com

The website of Dr. Michel Odent. He presents very scientific information. He has an archive of well-researched articles. He focuses on the life period with the highest adaptability and vulnerability to environmental factors—the period inside the womb.

Parenting

www.awakeparent.com

A newsletter in community work from the organization The Conscious Parenting Alliance.

www.freshstartafterdivorce.com

Begin again, no blame with help.

www.futurefamilies.org

A unique not-for-profit community association commenced in March 2007 by a group of Adelaide (South Australia) mums.

www.hpakids.org

Alliance for Holistic Family Health and Wellness.

www.mothering.com

Mothering Magazine—Earth-friendly, natural information.

www.quantumparenting.com

Spiritual and science parenting information.

Breastfeeding

www.thebreastsite.com

Everything you ever wanted to know about the breast but didn't know where to ask: health, surgery, breastfeeding, and resources.

www.breastfeeding.com

A site for mothers and nursing professionals who want support and advice.

www.llli.org

La Leche League-breastfeeding website.

www.promom.org

A site for the promotion of mother's milk.

RECOMMENDED READING
From Birth through Conscious Development

Gentle Birth Choices
By Barbara Harper, R.N. (Rochester, Vt.: Healing Arts Press, 2005)
Barbara Harper's book has been described as "one of the top ten books for pregnant women and their families" by the Lamaze International Organization. DVD included.

The Baby Book: Everything You Need to Know About Your Baby From Birth to Age Two
By Martha Sears and William Sears (Boston: Little, Brown, 2003)
This book is everything it says it is in the subtitle, and more. The classic "How to" book on what Sears has called "attachment" parenting. Thick as a phone book and crammed with information.

Magical Child
By Joseph Chilton Pearce (New York: Dutton, 1977)
This is my all time favorite child development book. It should be your first and primary. It is brilliant, thought provoking, and totally human. A carefully reasoned book that details the wisdom and magic of childhood and shows clearly why we must learn from our children. "Our very survival," he says, "depends on it."

Bradshaw On: The Family
By John Bradshaw (Deerfield Beach, Fla.: Health Communications, Inc., 1988)
Statistics tell us 96 percent of families are to some degree emotionally impaired. Our society is sick because our families are sick. And our families are sick because we are living by rules we never wrote: a life-affirming book that guides us out of our dysfunction to wholeness.

How Children Learn Series: Classics in Child Development
By John Holt (Cambridge, Mass.: Perseus Books, 1995)
A seminal classic, a must read for every parent.

And the Skylark Sings with Me: Adventures in Homeschooling and Community-Based Education

By David Albert (Gabriola Island, BC: New Society Publishing, 1999)

I consider this the definitive work on homeschooling. It shows what all parents can do to bring forth the best in their children and enjoy the riches of doing so—whether or not they attend school.

The Continuum Concept

By Jean Liedloff (Cambridge, Mass.: Perseus Books, 1985)

This book explores the author's two years among the Yaquana Indians of South America, a native culture living untouched by civilization. Liedloff's psychological insights about the parenting practices are penetrating, useful, and often hilarious.

Women's Bodies, Women's Wisdom: Creating Physical and Emotional Health and Healing

By Christiane Northrup (New York: Bantam Books, 1998)

This is, in my opinion, the best women's wellness book available: thorough and medically, psychologically, and spiritually enlightening.

The Psychology of Man's Possible Evolution

By P. D. Ouspensky (New York: Hedgehog Press, Inc., 1950)

This profound study of man's consciousness and possible evolution will awaken you in a way that you will find difficult to ignore.

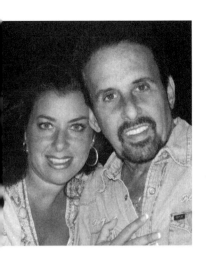

About the Authors

JEFFREY L. FINE, PH.D., an early pioneer in alternative health, preventive medicine, and holistic healing, has helped thousands of people in his thirty years of practice. He uses a directive approach to help clients solve their problems by stripping away their emotional clutter, and providing them with the tools they need to move confidently ahead in their lives. He gives clients a solid plan for how to cope with the most demanding days of their lives. He is a certified eating disorder specialist, an educator in Conscious Parenting, and has an interactive web-based therapy practice. He is the founder-director of the American Foundation for Conscious Parenting. The foundation is dedicated to spreading the teachings of healthy conception, pregnancy, birth, and parenting: working to educate and uplift underprivileged women and mothers and to bring this knowledge to schools, hospitals, and college educators through distribution of *The Art of Conscious Parenting* and seminars.

Dr. Fine is passionate about cultural change through promoting the new paradigm for conscious birth and parenting with new programs for healthy birth.

DALIT FINE earned a Master of Science degree in family counseling from City College at the City University of New York and a diploma in psychotherapy from the American Psychotherapy Association. She is a natural birth educator, a co-therapist with her husband, Dr. Fine, and a member of the American Psychotherapy Association. Both Jeffrey and Dalit are members of the Association for Pre- and Perinatal Psychology and Health.

Dalit is passionate about cultural change through promoting the new paradigm for conscious birth and mothering with unconditional love. Her mission is to awaken all women to the joy, ecstasy, and empowerment of natural birth and mothering.

To contact the authors go to
theNewParenting.com

Index

BOOKS OF RELATED INTEREST

Beyond the Icarus Factor
Releasing the Free Spirit of Boys
by Richard Hawley, Ph.D.

Children at Play
Using Waldorf Principles to Foster Childhood Development
by Heidi Britz-Crecelius

From Boys to Men
Spiritual Rites of Passage in an Indulgent Age
by Bret Stephenson

The Edison Gene
ADHD and the Gift of the Hunter Child
by Thom Hartmann

Birth without Violence
by Frédérick Leboyer, M.D.

Celebrating the Great Mother
A Handbook of Earth-Honoring Activities for Parents and Children
by Cait Johnson and Maura D. Shaw

Vaccinations: A Thoughtful Parent's Guide
How to Make Safe, Sensible Decisions about the Risks,
Benefits, and Alternatives
by Aviva Jill Romm

Walking the World in Wonder
A Children's Herbal
by Ellen Evert Hopman

INNER TRADITIONS • BEAR & COMPANY
P.O. Box 388
Rochester, VT 05767
1-800-246-8648
www.InnerTraditions.com

Or contact your local bookseller

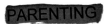